the
HEALTHY CARB
diabetes
COOKBOOK

Favorite Foods to Fit Your Meal Plan

Chef Jennifer Bucko, MCFE, &
Lara Rondinelli, RD, LDN, CDE

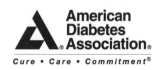

American
Diabetes
Association®

Cure • Care • Commitment®

Director, Book Publishing, **Robert Anthony**; *Managing Editor, Book Publishing*, **Abe Ogden**; *Editor*, **Greg Guthrie**; *Production Manager*, **Melissa Sprott**; *Composition*, **ADA**; *Cover Design*, **pixiedesign, LLC**; *Printer*, **Transcontinental Printing**.

Printed in Canada
3 5 7 9 10 8 6 4 2

♾ The paper in this publication meets the requirements of the ANSI Standard Z39.48-1992 (permanence of paper).

ADA titles may be purchased for business or promotional use or for special sales. To purchase more than 50 copies of this book at a discount, or for custom editions of this book with your logo, contact Jewelyn Morris, Special & Bulk Sales, at the address below, or at JMorris@diabetes.org or 703-299-2085.

For all other inquiries, please call 1-800-DIABETES.

American Diabetes Association
1701 North Beauregard Street
Alexandria, Virginia 22311

Library of Congress Cataloging-in-Publication Data

Bucko, Jennifer, 1974-
  Healthy carb diabetes cookbook / by Jennifer Bucko and Lara Rondinelli. – 1st ed.
     p. cm.
  Includes bibliographical references and index.
  ISBN 978-1-58040-291-0 (alk. paper)
  1. Diabetes–Diet therapy–Recipes. 2. Complex carbohydrate diet–Recipes I. Rondinelli, Lara M.,
1974- II. Title.

  RC662.B828 2007
  641.5'6314–dc22

                        2007042381

Contents

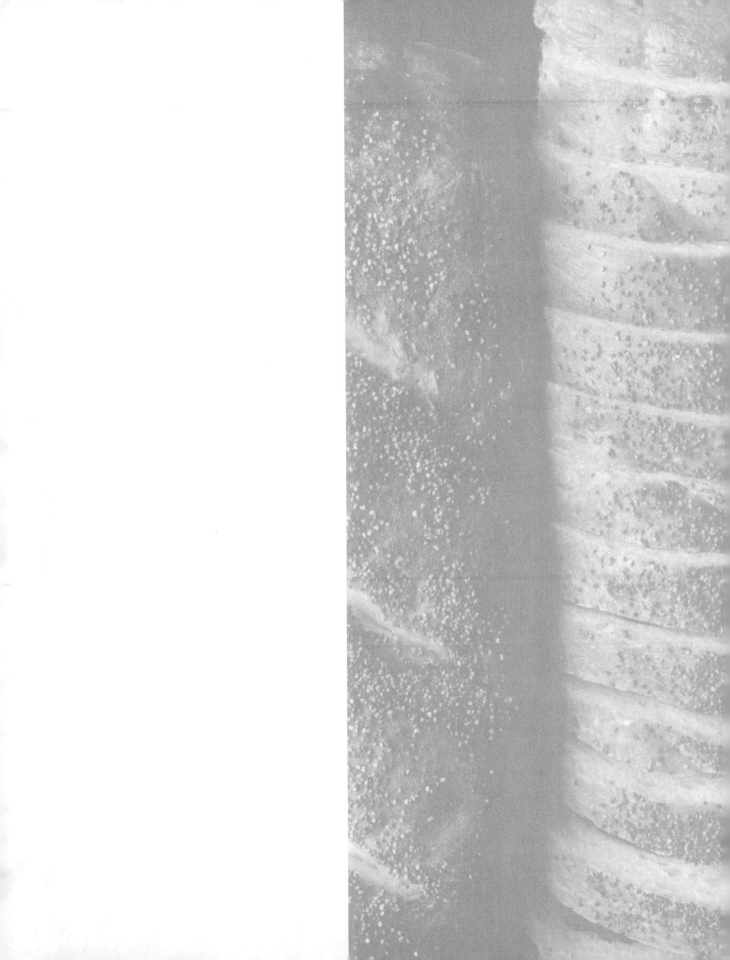

acknowledgments

FIRST, I must thank the many people who supported our first cookbook, *Healthy Calendar Diabetic Cooking*, because without that success, we wouldn't have been able to do this cookbook. The response to that book was amazing, and we have so many people to thank. Thank you to my family—my parents, Tom and Jane Rondinelli, and my sisters, Kari Mender and Jennifer Sebring—for being proud and great marketers. Thank you to my close friends, especially Draga Beckner, Meg Clendening, and Diane Zero, as well as the members of DECAADE. All of you were huge supporters, and I thank you.

For my growth in my diabetes education, I owe many thanks to my colleagues at Rush University Medical Center. Thank you to my boss, Dr. David Baldwin, for giving me the great opportunity to serve as Diabetes Center Coordinator. I have learned so much about every aspect of diabetes, and I'm very grateful for that. Thank you to my co-workers: Grace Villanueva, FNP, ND; Dr. Alexander Lurie; Dr. Arati Wagh; and Dr. Sharon Lahiri. Thanks for creating such a nice teaching and work environment. Thank you also to the Robert Morris College of Culinary Arts, especially to Nancy Rotunno, Dean and Executive Director, for supporting our efforts. Thank you to Brad Hindsley and Maegen Neal, culinary students, for all of your hard work and many hours spent on the recipes. Brad, I know you will make a wonderful chef; Maegen, you will make a great dietitian. While I was writing this book, a few of you helped when I especially needed it. Thank you, Jane Rondinelli, Jennifer Sebring, Megan Clendening, and Ann Marie Vidal.

Thank you to the many people at the American Diabetes Association for making this book possible. Thank you, Robert Anthony, Director of Book Publishing, for this great opportunity. Thanks to our editor, Greg Guthrie, for all of your hard work. Once again, huge thanks go to Madelyn Wheeler for doing a tremendous job on the nutrition analysis of the recipes. Thank you for all your feedback and your great attention to detail.

Thank you, Jared Hamilton, for making me laugh every single day that we are together and for being such a great taste tester. Thank you for your constant love and support and for sharing my excitement for food and this cookbook. I look forward to enjoying many more meals with you.

Thank you to my co-author and best friend, Jennifer Bucko, for another great project. It was fun as always. Not only are you an excellent chef and teacher, but also one of the dearest friends a person could ask for. Thank you for 21 years of wonderful friendship.

Finally, thank you again to all my patients with diabetes who continue to inspire me every day. I hope this cookbook helps prove that healthy eating does not have to be boring, tasteless, and complicated, but rather it shows that healthy eating and cooking can be quick, easy, and flavorful. Enjoy!

Lara Rondinelli
RD, LDN, CDE

• • •

MANY thanks to all of the people who helped make this book a reality, especially to my beloved, Michael Lamplough, who taste tested almost every recipe and put up with many, many piles of dishes. You, your love, and your support mean the world to me.

Thank you to my best friend and co-author, Lara Rondinelli, who is one of the most amazing people I know. Your skill, knowledge, dedication, and friendship are incredible, and I can't imagine working on a project like this with anyone else. Thanks for everything you always do for me.

Thank you to all of the staff and students at the Robert Morris College Institute of Culinary Arts, especially to Nancy Rotunno, Dean and Executive Director; Amy Keck, Director of Purchasing; and all of my fellow faculty members. Also, thank you to my students, Brad Hindsley and Maegen Neal, for all of your hard work on inputting the recipes. To all of you at RMC, your help, support, and enthusiasm helped us get this book done.

Many thanks to the staff at the American Diabetes Association, especially to Robert Anthony, Director of Book Publishing; Greg Guthrie, our fantastic editor; and Madelyn Wheeler, for her nutrition analysis of the recipes. We are grateful to you.

To the Bucko, Lamplough, and McKenzie families, thank you for your love, support, recipe ideas, taste testing, and senses of humor, all of which helped us create this book. A special thanks to my mom, Judy Bucko, who is a wonderful and talented woman and my number one cheerleader. And, as always, thanks go to my dad, Jack Bucko, who even though he isn't with us anymore is a part of every single thing I do.

Lastly, to everyone who has diabetes, I thank you for your inspiration and your desire to be healthy. I hope this book helps you and that you enjoy the food and a long healthy life. Eat well.

Chef Jennifer Bucko
MCFE

• • •

ACCORDING to the American Diabetes Association, people with diabetes are encouraged to choose a variety of fiber-containing foods (such as fruits, vegetables, and legumes), fiber-rich cereals, and whole-grain products. Whole grains have been a hot topic ever since the 2005 release of the USDA Dietary Guidelines, which recommended that of the grains eaten, at least one-half should come from whole-grain foods. According to these guidelines, eating at least three servings of whole grains per day may reduce the risk of several chronic diseases, including heart disease, cancer, and diabetes, and may also help with weight loss. Whole grains have always been known to provide dietary fiber, but they also provide vitamins, minerals, and antioxidants that are not found in other foods.

But the big question is: what exactly is a whole grain?

Whole grains consist of the entire grain seed, usually called the kernel. The kernel has three components: bran, germ, and endosperm. All grains are whole grains when they are first harvested, and if they keep these three components in the final food product, they qualify as a whole grain.

Common Whole-Grain Foods in the U.S.

Whole wheat	Whole-grain rye
Whole oats/oatmeal	Whole-grain barley
Whole-grain corn	Buckwheat
Popcorn	Bulgur
Brown rice	Quinoa
Wild rice	

Source: Agriculture Research Service Database for CSFII 1994–1996.

You can't tell whether a food is whole grain by its color. Just because bread is brown in color does not necessarily mean that it is whole grain. The only way to be truly sure about whether a food is whole grain is by reading food labels, specifically the ingredients list on the packaging. For many whole-grain products, the word "whole" or "whole grain" will appear before the grain ingredient's name. The whole grain should also be the first ingredient listed in the ingredient list. For example, whole-wheat flour can be the first ingredient for whole-grain bread, but if "wheat flour" or "enriched flour" is the first ingredient, then the food is not whole grain.

The food industry responded to the Dietary Guidelines and introduced a variety of whole-grain products, including whole-grain cereals, whole-wheat pastas, whole-wheat English muffins and bagels, whole-wheat pizza crusts, whole-grain crackers, whole-wheat tortillas, and many more. Most of these products are available at any grocery store in your local area and many were used in this cookbook.

In addition to eating whole-grain foods, people with diabetes should consume other healthy carbohydrates.

- Fresh fruit is a great source of fiber, vitamins, and minerals. Fruit should be eaten daily and counted toward your daily total carbohydrate intake.
- Choose low-fat or fat-free dairy products, such as nonfat milk and light yogurt. These provide calcium, which is important for bone health. They should be eaten daily and counted toward total carbohydrate intake.
- Lean protein sources, such as chicken breast, turkey, fish, and lean beef and pork, should be selected over higher-fat foods. Lean protein foods do not raise blood glucose levels and are lower in saturated fat, which is important for heart health.
- People with diabetes should limit their intake of saturated and trans-fats and instead choose monounsaturated and polyunsaturated fats, such as olive oil, canola oil, nuts, almonds, seeds, and avocados, because they are better for your heart.
- Low-carbohydrate vegetables, such as greens, spinach, broccoli, cauliflower, zucchini, lettuce, Brussels sprouts, and green beans, should be eaten daily and should take up half of your dinner plate. These foods are low in fat, calories, and carbohydrates and have a minimal effect on blood glucose levels.

This cookbook contains quick and tasty recipes that use only the healthiest carbohydrate foods: whole grains, fruit, vegetables, and low-fat dairy products, along with lean protein sources and heart-healthy fats. The recipes use a combination of foods to produce mouthwatering, high-fiber, low-fat meals that can be prepared in a snap. Do you find that you're often asking what to eat from one day to the next? If so, then this book is the tool to help you answer that question tonight and every night. These meals are healthy, can be easily prepared, and do not require special trips to health food stores. Most of the ingredients for these recipes can be found in your local grocery store. This book is designed for the everyday person trying to put quick and healthy meals together day after day.

After the release of our first cookbook, *Healthy Calendar Diabetic Cooking*, which provided dinner recipes for the entire year, people requested even more healthy recipes. So this book provides breakfast, lunch, dinner, side dishes, and dessert recipes. You will see that healthy eating can be a part of every delicious meal and dessert. Enjoy!

breakfast

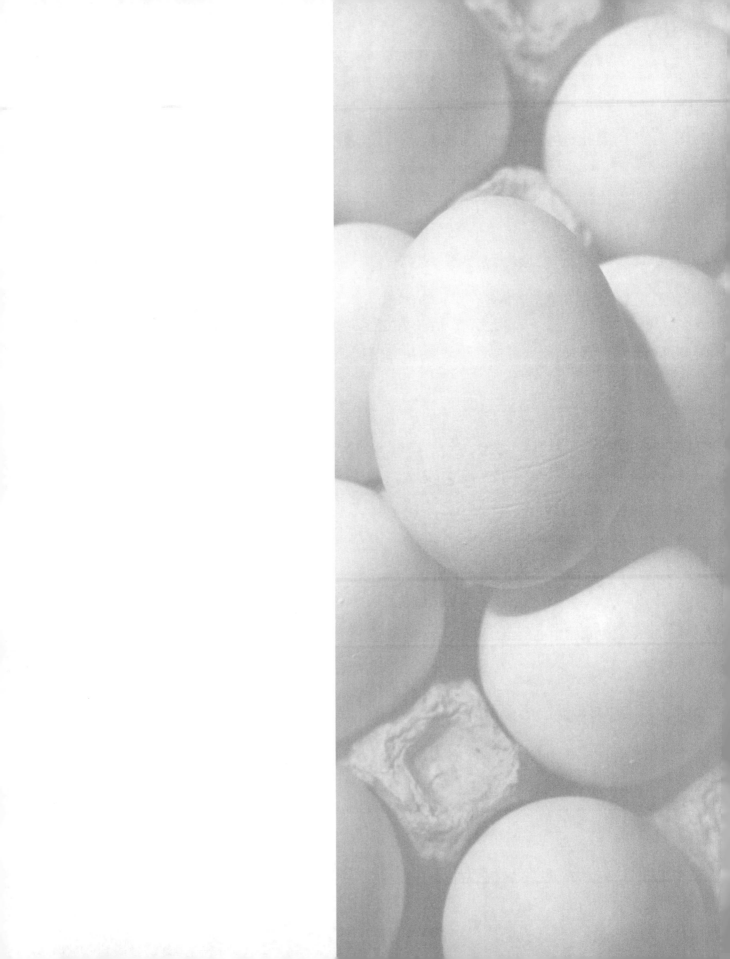

APPLE PECAN STUFFED FRENCH TOAST

Serves 6 • Serving Size: 1/2 sandwich • Prep Time: 20 minutes

Cooking spray

2 medium Granny Smith apples, peeled, cored, and thinly sliced

3/4 cup low-fat ricotta cheese

1/4 cup chopped pecans

1/2 cup Splenda, divided

1 1/2 tsp ground cinnamon, divided

1 cup egg substitute

1 cup fat-free half-and-half

12 slices whole-wheat bread

Sugar-free syrup (*optional*)

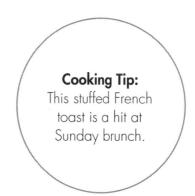

Cooking Tip:
This stuffed French toast is a hit at Sunday brunch.

1. Coat a medium nonstick sauté pan with cooking spray. Sauté apples until they begin to soften, about 10 minutes. Set aside to cool.

2. In a small mixing bowl, combine ricotta, pecans, 1/4 cup Splenda, and 1/2 tsp cinnamon. Fold in cooled apples.

3. In a medium bowl, whisk together egg substitute, fat-free half-and-half, remaining Splenda, and remaining cinnamon.

4. Divide the cheese mixture into six equal portions. Spread one slice of bread with 1/6 of cheese mixture. Top with another slice of bread. Repeat to make six sandwiches.

5. Coat a large nonstick skillet with cooking spray. Heat over medium heat. Dip each sandwich in egg mixture and cook for 3–4 minutes per side until golden brown. Remove from heat and cut in half diagonally.

6. Serve with sugar-free syrup, if desired.

Exchanges/Choices
1 Starch
1 Lean Meat
1/2 Fat

Calories	140
Calories from Fat	30
Total Fat	3.5 g
Saturated Fat	1 g
Trans Fat	0 g
Cholesterol	5 mg
Sodium	230 mg
Total Carbohydrate	19 g
Dietary Fiber	3 g
Sugars	7 g
Protein	8 g

BERRY WAFFLES

Serves 6 • Serving Size: 1 waffle • Prep Time: 5 minutes

1 cup strawberries, sliced

1 cup blueberries

1 cup raspberries

3 Tbsp Splenda

6 low-fat, whole-grain frozen waffles, toasted

2 Tbsp low-sugar, strawberry jelly

6 Tbsp light whipped topping

1. In a medium bowl, stir together all of the berries and the Splenda.

2. Spread each toasted waffle with 1 tsp jelly and top with 1/2 cup berry mixture and 1 Tbsp whipped topping.

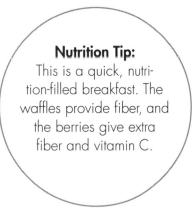

Nutrition Tip:
This is a quick, nutrition-filled breakfast. The waffles provide fiber, and the berries give extra fiber and vitamin C.

Exchanges/Choices
1 Starch
1/2 Fruit

Calories 125
  Calories from Fat.....20
Total Fat ....2 g
  Saturated Fat ....0.8 g
  Trans Fat ....0 g
Cholesterol ....0 mg
Sodium ....215 mg
Total Carbohydrate ....26 g
  Dietary Fiber ....4 g
  Sugars ....9 g
Protein......................3 g

BLUEBERRY MUFFINS

Serves 10 • Serving Size: 1 muffin • Prep Time: 20 minutes

Cooking spray

1 1/2 cups old-fashioned rolled oats

1 cup bran flakes, crushed

1/2 cup whole-wheat flour

1/4 cup Splenda Brown Sugar Blend

2 tsp ground cinnamon

1 tsp baking powder

1 tsp baking soda

1/2 tsp salt

1 1/3 cups low-fat buttermilk

1/2 cup fat-free sour cream

1/4 cup canola oil

1 large egg

1 tsp vanilla

2 cups frozen blueberries

1 Tbsp whole-wheat flour

1. Preheat oven to 400°F. Line a muffin pan with 12 paper liners and spray lightly with cooking spray.

2. In a large bowl, combine oats, bran flakes, whole-wheat flour, Splenda Brown Sugar Blend, cinnamon, baking powder, baking soda, and salt. Mix well.

3. In a medium bowl, whisk together buttermilk, sour cream, oil, egg, and vanilla. Add this mixture to flour mixture, gently stirring until moist; do not overmix.

4. In a small bowl toss blueberries with 1 Tbsp whole-wheat flour. Gently fold blueberries into muffin batter.

5. Spoon about 1/2 cup batter into each muffin cup. Bake for 20 minutes or until a toothpick inserted in the center comes out clean. Cool on a wire rack.

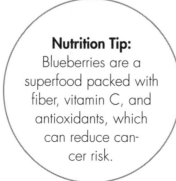

Nutrition Tip:
Blueberries are a superfood packed with fiber, vitamin C, and antioxidants, which can reduce cancer risk.

Exchanges/Choices
2 Carbohydrate
1 1/2 Fat

Calories 200
   Calories from Fat.....65
Total Fat....................7 g
   Saturated Fat.............0.9 g
   Trans Fat ....0 g
Cholesterol ....25 mg
Sodium ....370 mg
Total Carbohydrate....28 g
   Dietary Fiber ....4 g
   Sugars ....10 g
Protein......................6 g

BREAKFAST BURRITO

Serves 4 • Serving Size: 1 burrito • Prep Time: 10 minutes

3 Tbsp jalapeño pepper, seeded and finely chopped

1 large tomato, seeded and diced

1/4 cup green onion, chopped

1/4 cup reduced-fat, shredded cheddar cheese

3 whole eggs

4 egg whites

1/8 tsp salt (*optional*)

1/8 tsp ground black pepper

Cooking spray

4 whole-wheat tortillas, warmed*

4 Tbsp salsa

Cooking Tip:
If you prefer to have your burritos less spicy, substitute green bell pepper for jalapeño pepper.

1. In a medium bowl, combine the first eight ingredients (including optional salt). Coat a nonstick skillet with cooking spray and heat over medium-high heat. Add egg mixture. Cook, without stirring, until egg mixture begins to set on the bottom. Draw a spatula across the bottom of the pan to form large curds. Continue cooking until egg mixture is thick but still moist; do not stir constantly.

2. Fill one tortilla with a portion of the egg mixture and 1 Tbsp salsa. Fold the sides of the tortilla in and then up from the bottom to form a burrito.

3. Repeat process for the remaining three burritos.

Exchanges/Choices
2 Starch
1 Vegetable
1 Lean Meat
1 Fat

Calories	275
Calories from Fat	80
Total Fat	9 g
Saturated Fat	2.4 g
Trans Fat	0 g
Cholesterol	165 mg
Sodium	660 mg
Total Carbohydrate	33 g
Dietary Fiber	5 g
Sugars	4 g
Protein	15 g

Each tortilla should have 30 g carbohydrate and 4 g dietary fiber per serving.

BREAKFAST COOKIE

Serves 24 • Serving Size: 1 cookie • Prep Time: 20 minutes

Cooking spray

1/2 cup Splenda Brown Sugar Blend

1/2 cup canola oil

2 egg whites

1 tsp vanilla

1/2 cup peanut butter

2 medium ripe bananas, mashed

1 cup whole-wheat flour

2 cups old-fashioned rolled oats

1/4 cup milled flaxseed

3/4 cup bran flakes, crushed

1 1/2 tsp ground cinnamon

1/2 tsp baking soda

1/2 tsp salt (*optional*)

1. Preheat oven to 350°F. Spray a large baking sheet with cooking spray or line with parchment paper.

2. In a medium bowl, mix together Splenda Brown Sugar Blend and oil. Add egg whites and vanilla, and beat until smooth. Add peanut butter and bananas, and beat well.

3. In a large bowl, combine flour, oats, flaxseed, bran flakes, cinnamon, baking soda, and salt (optional). Make a well in the center of the dry ingredients and pour in the egg mixture. Fold wet ingredients into dry ingredients until batter is incorporated.

4. Scoop cookies into two-inch balls and place on cookie sheet. Bake 8–10 minutes or until slightly golden on bottom. Cool on wire rack.

Cooking Tip:
Baking with whole-wheat flour can be a challenge because using too much can make baked foods tough, but using oats, flaxseed, or bran flakes helps make tender, delicious, and filling cookies.

Exchanges/Choices
1 Carbohydrate
1 1/2 Fat

Calories	155
Calories from Fat	70
Total Fat	8 g
Saturated Fat	1 g
Trans Fat	0 g
Cholesterol	0 mg
Sodium	75 mg
Total Carbohydrate	17 g
Dietary Fiber	3 g
Sugars	6 g
Protein	4 g

BREAKFAST SHAKE

Serves 2 • Serving Size: 1 cup • Prep Time: 5 minutes

1 cup frozen mixed berries (strawberries, blueberries, raspberries)

1 6-oz container light, nonfat berry yogurt

1/4 cup nonfat milk

1 Tbsp Splenda

1. Place all ingredients in a blender.

2. Blend until smooth.

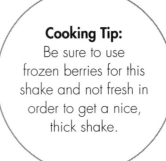

Cooking Tip:
Be sure to use
frozen berries for this
shake and not fresh in
order to get a nice,
thick shake.

Exchanges/Choices
1/2 Fruit
1 Fat-Free Milk

Calories 80
  Calories from Fat.......0
Total Fat ....0 g
  Saturated Fat ....0 g
  Trans Fat ....0 g
Cholesterol ....0 mg
Sodium ....60 mg
Total Carbohydrate ....17 g
  Dietary Fiber ....1 g
  Sugars ....13 g
Protein ....4 g

CINNAMON OATMEAL WITH WALNUTS

Serves 4 • Serving Size: 1/2 cup • Prep Time: 5 minutes

2 cups dry old-fashioned rolled oats

4 cups water

4 Tbsp walnuts, chopped and toasted

4 tsp ground cinnamon

4 tsp Splenda Brown Sugar Blend

1 Tbsp Splenda

1. In a small pan, cook oatmeal according to package instructions.

2. Add remaining ingredients and mix well.

Nutrition Tip:
Oatmeal is a quick, high-fiber breakfast, and the walnuts and Splenda Brown Sugar Blend make it delicious.

Exchanges/Choices
2 Starch
1 1/2 Fat

Calories	230
Calories from Fat	70
Total Fat	8 g
Saturated Fat	0.9 g
Trans Fat	0 g
Cholesterol	0 mg
Sodium	15 mg
Total Carbohydrate	34 g
Dietary Fiber	6 g
Sugars	5 g
Protein	8 g

the healthy carb diabetes cookbook

EGG SANDWICH

Serves 4 • Serving Size: 1 sandwich • Prep Time: 10 minutes

Cooking spray

4 slices Canadian bacon

1 cup egg substitute

1/8 tsp ground black pepper

4 whole-wheat English muffins, split and toasted

4 (1-oz) slices fat-free American cheese

1. Coat a medium skillet with cooking spray. Add Canadian bacon. Cook over medium heat 1–2 minutes on each side. Remove from pan.

2. In a medium bowl, beat egg substitute and black pepper with a wire whisk until well blended; pour into skillet. Cook until egg substitute is almost set; draw a spatula across the pan to form large curds. Cook an additional 4–5 minutes, or until eggs are firm but still moist, stirring occasionally.

3. Spoon about 1/4 of egg mixture over one English muffin half; top with 1 slice Canadian bacon, 1 slice cheese, and other English muffin half. Repeat for remaining three sandwiches.

Exchanges/Choices
2 Starch
2 Lean Meat

Calories 245
   Calories from Fat.....30
Total Fat ....3.5 g
   Saturated Fat.............0.9 g
   Trans Fat ....0 g
Cholesterol ....20 mg
Sodium ....1150 mg
Total Carbohydrate ....31 g
   Dietary Fiber ....4 g
   Sugars ....8 g
Protein ....24 g

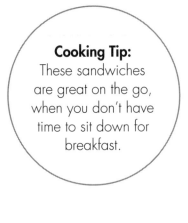

Cooking Tip:
These sandwiches are great on the go, when you don't have time to sit down for breakfast.

This recipe is high in sodium.

FRENCH TOAST MUFFINS

Serves 6 • Serving Size: 1 muffin • Prep Time: 10 minutes

Cooking spray
1 1/2 cups egg substitute
1/2 cup fat-free half-and-half
1 tsp ground cinnamon
3 Tbsp Splenda
2 Tbsp milled flaxseed
1 tsp vanilla
6 slices whole-wheat bread, cut into chunks

Nutrition Tip:
Find flaxseed in the baking aisle of grocery stores. The American Heart Association recommends eating flaxseed because it contains alpha-linolenic acid and protects against heart disease.

1. Preheat oven to 400°F.

2. Spray muffin pan with cooking spray.

3. In a medium bowl, whisk together egg substitute, fat-free half-and-half, cinnamon, Splenda, flaxseed, and vanilla.

4. Gently fold bread into egg mixture, let sit 5 minutes to soak.

5. Divide mixture evenly among six muffin cups; overfilling slightly.

6. Bake for 25 minutes or until puffed and set. Serve immediately and with sugar-free syrup if desired.

Exchanges/Choices
1 Starch
1 Lean Meat

Calories	140
Calories from Fat	20
Total Fat	2.5 g
Saturated Fat	0.5 g
Trans Fat	0 g
Cholesterol	0 mg
Sodium	270 mg
Total Carbohydrate	17 g
Dietary Fiber	3 g
Sugars	4 g
Protein	11 g

the healthy carb diabetes cookbook

LOX BAGEL SANDWICH

Serves 4 • Serving Size: 1 bagel sandwich • Prep Time: 10 minutes

4 small whole-wheat bagels (30 grams carbohydrate per bagel), cut in half

2 Tbsp light mayonnaise

4 oz smoked salmon (4 1-oz slices)

4 slices tomato

4 lettuce leaves

8 cucumber slices

1/2 red onion, sliced

1. Toast bagels. Add 1/2 Tbsp mayonnaise to one side of bagel.

2. Top mayonnaise with one slice smoked salmon, one tomato slice, one lettuce leaf, 2 cucumber slices, and red onion slices. Top with remaining bagel half. Repeat for remaining three sandwiches.

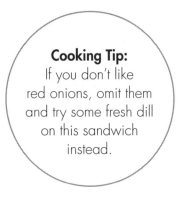

Cooking Tip:
If you don't like red onions, omit them and try some fresh dill on this sandwich instead.

Exchanges/Choices	
2 Starch	
1 Vegetable	
1 Lean Meat	

Calories	220
Calories from Fat	40
Total Fat	4.5 g
Saturated Fat	0.8 g
Trans Fat	0 g
Cholesterol	10 mg
Sodium	540 mg
Total Carbohydrate	34 g
Dietary Fiber	4 g
Sugars	7 g
Protein	13 g

MINI BREAKFAST PIZZA

Serves 6 • Serving Size: 1 pizza • Prep Time: 20 minutes

1/4 cup Splenda

1/2 tsp ground cinnamon

3 whole-wheat pita pockets

Cooking spray

1 cup prepared sugar-free, fat-free vanilla
   pudding

1 oz light cream cheese

1 cup strawberries, sliced

1 cup blueberries

2 kiwi fruit, peeled and sliced

Cooking Tip:
Different fruit can
be substituted here if
desired; for example,
peaches, apples, or
raspberries could
also be used.

1. Preheat oven to 350°F.

2. In a small bowl mix together the Splenda and cinnamon.

3. Split the pitas in half, making two round halves for each individual pita.

4. Place pitas on baking sheet cut side up and spray each pita with cooking spray. Sprinkle each pita evenly with the cinnamon and Splenda mixture. Bake pitas for 10 minutes. Cool.

5. In a small bowl, blend pudding and cream cheese together until smooth.

6. Spread 2 Tbsp pudding mixture on each pita.

7. Top each pita with equal amounts of fresh berries and kiwi slices.

Exchanges/Choices	
1 Starch	
1/2 Fruit	
1/2 Carbohydrate	
1/2 Fat	
Calories	145
Calories from Fat	20
Total Fat	2 g
Saturated Fat	0.8 g
Trans Fat	0 g
Cholesterol	5 mg
Sodium	390 mg
Total Carbohydrate	30 g
Dietary Fiber	4 g
Sugars	7 g
Protein	4 g

OVERNIGHT APPLE FRENCH TOAST

Serves 6 • Serving Size: 1 slice bread, 1 scoop apple • Prep Time: 15 minutes

1/3 cup Splenda Brown Sugar Blend

3 Tbsp light trans-fat-free margarine

2 Tbsp sugar-free syrup

3 Granny Smith apples, peeled, cored, and sliced

1/2 cup nonfat milk

1 whole egg

4 egg whites

1 tsp ground cinnamon

1 tsp vanilla

6 slices whole-wheat bread

Cooking Tip:
This dish is great when you are having guests over and don't want to spend your morning fixing breakfast. Just put this dish in the oven in the morning and your guests will awaken to the wonderful aroma of apples and cinnamon.

1. In a small saucepan over medium heat cook Splenda Brown Sugar Blend, margarine, and syrup until it thickens, about 5–7 minutes.

2. Pour mixture into a 9 × 13-inch glass baking dish and arrange sliced apples on top.

3. In a small bowl mix milk, egg, egg whites, cinnamon, and vanilla. Dip each slice of bread into milk mixture. Place dipped bread slices over apples.

4. Cover and refrigerate overnight. Remove from refrigerator 30 minutes before baking.

5. Preheat oven to 350°F. Bake for 30–35 minutes.

Exchanges/Choices
2 Carbohydrate
1 Lean Meat
1/2 Fat

Calories 205
    Calories from Fat.....40
Total Fat ....4.5 g
    Saturated Fat ....1.2 g
    Trans Fat ....0 g
Cholesterol ....35 mg
Sodium ....240 mg
Total Carbohydrate ....33 g
    Dietary Fiber ....3 g
    Sugars ....22 g
Protein ....8 g

PEANUT BUTTER GRANOLA

Serves 11 • Serving Size: 1/2 cup • Prep Time: 15 minutes

Cooking spray

3 cups old-fashioned rolled oats

1 cup Cheerios cereal

1/3 cup oat bran

1/4 cup walnuts, finely chopped

2 tsp ground cinnamon

1/4 cup peanut butter

1/3 cup applesauce

2 Tbsp honey

1 Tbsp Splenda Brown Sugar Blend

Nutrition Tip:
When served over light yogurt and berries, this granola offers a great power-packed breakfast.

1. Preheat oven to 300°F. Coat a 9 × 13-inch baking dish with cooking spray.

2. In a large bowl, combine oats, Cheerios, oat bran, walnuts, and cinnamon.

3. Melt peanut butter in a medium saucepan over medium heat. Add applesauce, honey, and Splenda Brown Sugar Blend. Bring to a boil. Cook for 1 minute, stirring frequently.

4. Pour applesauce mixture over oat mixture, stirring to coat. Pour mixture into baking dish. Bake for 25–30 minutes.

Exchanges/Choices
1 Starch
1/2 Carbohydrate
1 Fat

Calories 175
  Calories from Fat 65
Total Fat .... 7 g
  Saturated Fat .... 1.1 g
  Trans Fat .... 0 g
Cholesterol .... 0 mg
Sodium .... 50 mg
Total Carbohydrate .... 26 g
  Dietary Fiber .... 4 g
  Sugars .... 6 g
Protein .... 6 g

PUMPKIN PIE FRENCH TOAST

Serves 10 • Serving Size: 1 piece • Prep Time: 5 minutes

3/4 cup egg substitute

1 cup fat-free half-and-half

1 15-oz can pure pumpkin

1 Tbsp pumpkin pie spice

1 tsp ground cinnamon

1/2 cup Splenda

Cooking spray

10 whole-wheat bread slices

10 tsp light whipped topping

Ground nutmeg for garnish

1. In a medium bowl, whisk together egg substitute, fat-free half-and-half, pumpkin, pumpkin pie spice, cinnamon, and Splenda.

2. Coat a large nonstick skillet with cooking spray over medium heat.

3. Dip each bread slice into batter and then cook on each side for 3–4 minutes or until golden brown, working in batches.

4. Serve with a spoonful of whipped topping and a light dusting of nutmeg.

Exchanges/Choices
1 Starch
1/2 Carbohydrate

Calories	115
Calories from Fat	15
Total Fat	1.5 g
Saturated Fat	0.7 g
Trans Fat	0 g
Cholesterol	0 mg
Sodium	195 mg
Total Carbohydrate	20 g
Dietary Fiber	3 g
Sugars	6 g
Protein	7 g

Cooking Tip:
Be sure to buy 100% pure pumpkin in the can and not pumpkin pie filling for this decadent breakfast.

SPINACH, BACON, AND MUSHROOM MINI EGG SOUFFLÉ

Serves 8 • Serving Size: 1 mini-egg soufflé • Prep Time: 10 minutes

8 muffin paper liners
Cooking spray
5 slices turkey bacon, diced
1 cup mushrooms, diced
1 cup egg substitute
10 oz frozen spinach, thawed and drained
1/4 cup reduced-fat feta cheese, crumbled
1/4 tsp salt (*optional*)
1/8 tsp ground black pepper

1. Preheat oven to 350°F. Line a muffin pan with 8 paper liners and coat lightly with cooking spray.

2. In a medium pan, sauté bacon until crisp, add mushrooms, and cook for an additional 4–5 minutes or until liquid is reduced. Set aside to cool.

3. In a medium bowl, add egg substitute and all remaining ingredients and mix well. Stir in bacon and mushrooms to combine.

4. Pour 1/4 cup egg mixture into each lined muffin tin and bake for 20 minutes.

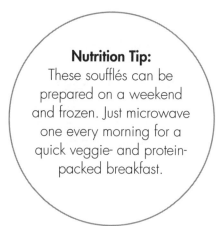

Nutrition Tip:
These soufflés can be prepared on a weekend and frozen. Just microwave one every morning for a quick veggie- and protein-packed breakfast.

Exchanges/Choices
1 Lean Meat

Calories	55
Calories from Fat	20
Total Fat	2.5 g
Saturated Fat	0.9 g
Trans Fat	0 g
Cholesterol	10 mg
Sodium	250 mg
Total Carbohydrate	2 g
Dietary Fiber	1 g
Sugars	1 g
Protein	7 g

STRAWBERRY OAT MUFFINS

Serves 12 • Serving Size: 1 muffin • Prep Time: 10 minutes

12 muffin paper liners

Cooking spray

1 1/4 cup plus 1 Tbsp old-fashioned rolled oats (reserve 1 Tbsp)

3/4 cup whole-wheat flour

2 Tbsp Splenda Sugar Blend for Baking

2 Tbsp Splenda Brown Sugar Blend

1 1/2 tsp baking powder

1/2 tsp salt (*optional*)

1 cup nonfat milk

3 Tbsp canola oil

1 large egg

1 tsp vanilla

6 Tbsp low-sugar strawberry preserves

1. Preheat oven to 375°F. Line a muffin pan with 12 paper liners and spray lightly with cooking spray.

2. In a large bowl combine the oats, whole-wheat flour, Splenda Sugar Blend for Baking, Splenda Brown Sugar Blend, baking powder, and salt (optional). Mix well.

3. In a medium bowl whisk together the milk, oil, egg, and vanilla.

4. Make a well in the center of dry ingredients. Add milk (wet ingredients) mixture and stir until moist; do not overmix.

Cooking Tip:
Try substituting low-sugar apricot or apple jelly for the strawberry or try a mix of flavors for a nice surprise.

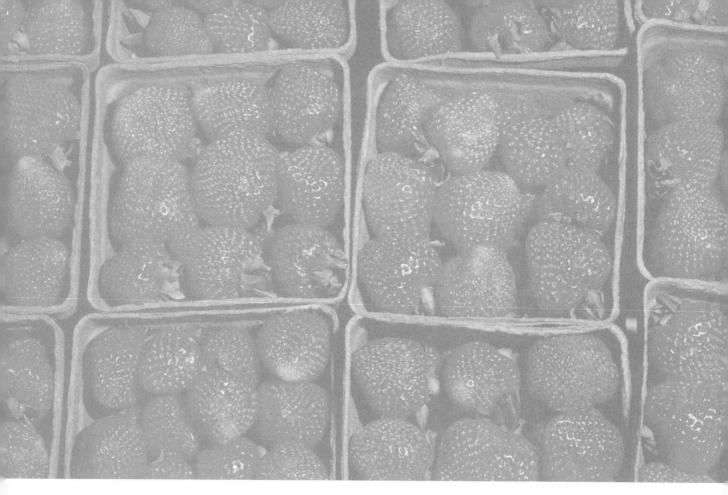

5. Spoon about 1 Tbsp batter into each muffin cup. Spoon 1 tsp strawberry preserves into center of muffin cup, but do not spread. Spoon remaining batter over strawberry preserves, dividing evenly.

6. Sprinkle each filled muffin cup with reserved 1 Tbsp oats.

7. Bake 20–25 minutes. Cool completely on wire rack.

Exchanges/Choices		
1 1/2 Carbohydrate		
1/2 Fat		

Calories	135
Calories from Fat	40
Total Fat	4.5 g
Saturated Fat	0.5 g
Trans Fat	0 g
Cholesterol	20 mg
Sodium	65 mg
Total Carbohydrate	20 g
Dietary Fiber	2 g
Sugars	8 g
Protein	4 g

TURKEY SAUSAGE AND EGG CASSEROLE

Serves 10 • Serving Size: 1/10th recipe • Prep Time: 10 minutes

Cooking spray

2 cups nonfat milk

1/2 cup green onions, chopped

1/2 tsp dry mustard

1/4 tsp salt (*optional*)

1/4 tsp ground black pepper

16 oz egg substitute

4 slices whole-wheat bread, cut into 1/2-inch cubes

3 precooked turkey breakfast sausage patties, diced

1/4 cup reduced-fat, shredded cheddar cheese

1. Preheat oven to 350°F. Coat a 9 × 13-inch baking dish with cooking spray.

2. In a medium bowl, whisk together nonfat milk, green onions, dry mustard, salt (optional), pepper, and egg substitute.

3. Place bread cubes and sausage on the bottom of the baking dish, pour egg mixture evenly over bread and sausage. Top with cheddar cheese.

4. Cover pan with aluminum foil and bake for 20 minutes. Remove foil and bake for an additional 40 minutes.

Exchanges/Choices
1/2 Carbohydrate
2 Lean Meat

Calories	110
Calories from Fat	20
Total Fat	2.5 g
Saturated Fat	0.9 g
Trans Fat	0 g
Cholesterol	15 mg
Sodium	295 mg
Total Carbohydrate	8 g
Dietary Fiber	1 g
Sugars	4 g
Protein	13 g

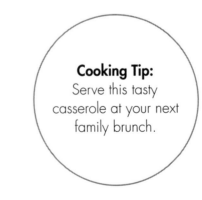

Cooking Tip:
Serve this tasty casserole at your next family brunch.

VEGGIE OMELET

Serves 4 • Serving Size: 1 omelet • Prep Time: 15 minutes

Cooking spray
1 small green bell pepper, diced
1 small onion, diced
1 small zucchini, diced
1 small tomato, diced
2 cups egg substitute
1/2 cup fat-free half-and-half
1/4 tsp salt (*optional*)
1/8 tsp ground black pepper
1/2 cup reduced-fat, shredded cheddar cheese

Cooking Tip:
Make sure to use a good nonstick pan or omelet pan, so it is easy to fold and flip your omelet.

1. Spray a large sauté pan with cooking spray over medium heat.

2. Sauté bell pepper, onion, and zucchini until onions are clear and zucchini is tender. Add tomatoes and sauté for 2 more minutes.

3. Remove vegetables from heat and set aside to cool.

4. In a medium bowl, whisk together egg substitute, fat-free half-and-half, salt (optional), and pepper.

5. Spray a small nonstick sauté pan or omelet pan with cooking spray and place over medium heat.

6. Pour 1/2 cup egg mixture into pan and let the omelet start to set. Add 1/4 cup vegetable mixture and 2 Tbsp of cheese to one side of the omelet. Fold the other side over the vegetables and cheese. Flip the omelet to finish cooking and serve.

7. Repeat to make four omelets.

Exchanges/Choices
1/2 Carbohydrate
1 Vegetable
2 Lean Meat

Calories	145
Calories from Fat.....	30
Total Fat	3.5 g
Saturated Fat	2.1 g
Trans Fat	0 g
Cholesterol	10 mg
Sodium	380 mg
Total Carbohydrate	11 g
Dietary Fiber	1 g
Sugars	6 g
Protein	17 g

WHOLE-WHEAT CINNAMON PANCAKES

Serves 10 • Serving Size: 1 pancake • Prep Time: 15 minutes

1/3 cup old-fashioned rolled oats

1/3 cup wheat germ

1 cup low-fat buttermilk

1 whole egg

2 egg whites

1 tsp vanilla

1 cup nonfat milk

1 cup whole-wheat flour

1 1/2 tsp baking powder

1 tsp baking soda

1/4 tsp salt (*optional*)

2 tsp ground cinnamon

1/3 cup Splenda

Cooking spray

1. In a medium bowl, combine oats, wheat germ, and buttermilk. Let stand until oats soften. Mix in egg, egg whites, vanilla, and nonfat milk.

2. In a large bowl, mix together whole-wheat flour, baking powder, baking soda, salt (optional), cinnamon, and Splenda.

3. Make a well in the center of the dry ingredients. Pour entire wet mixture into the well and fold together until completely incorporated.

4. Coat a griddle or nonstick skillet with cooking spray and heat over medium heat. Use 1/3 cup batter for each pancake and cook until brown on bottom and some bubbles begin to break around edges. Turn pancake over and cook until brown and slightly firm to the touch in the center.

5. Repeat procedure until all batter is gone.

Exchanges/Choices
1 Starch

Calories	100
Calories from Fat	15
Total Fat	1.5 g
Saturated Fat	0.4 g
Trans Fat	0 g
Cholesterol	25 mg
Sodium	240 mg
Total Carbohydrate	16 g
Dietary Fiber	2 g
Sugars	4 g
Protein	6 g

Cooking Tip:
These pancakes can be topped with bananas, blueberries, or mixed berries or served with sugar-free syrup.

YOGURT PARFAIT

Serves 4 • Serving Size: 1 parfait • Prep Time: 10 minutes

2 cups fat-free plain yogurt

1 Tbsp Splenda

1 1/2 cups assorted berries, fresh or frozen (*see tip*)

4 Tbsp sliced almonds, toasted

1. In a small bowl, combine yogurt and Splenda. In a parfait dish or fluted glass, layer 1/4 cup yogurt and 3 Tbsp berries. Repeat process once more, and top with 1 Tbsp toasted almonds.

2. Repeat this procedure for remaining three parfaits.

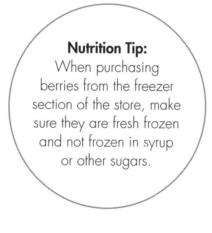

Nutrition Tip:
When purchasing berries from the freezer section of the store, make sure they are fresh frozen and not frozen in syrup or other sugars.

Exchanges/Choices
1/2 Fruit
1/2 Fat-Free Milk
1/2 Fat

Calories	115
Calories from Fat	25
Total Fat	3 g
Saturated Fat	0.4 g
Trans Fat	0 g
Cholesterol	10 mg
Sodium	80 mg
Total Carbohydrate	16 g
Dietary Fiber	3 g
Sugars	12 g
Protein	8 g

YOGURT WITH TOASTED ALMONDS AND JAM

Serves 4 • Serving Size: 1 cup • Prep Time: 5 minutes

4 cups fat-free, plain yogurt

1/4 cup Splenda

4 Tbsp low-sugar raspberry jam

4 Tbsp slivered almonds, toasted

In a medium bowl, combine yogurt and Splenda. Divide evenly among three small serving bowls. Dollop each bowl of yogurt with 1 Tbsp jam, and sprinkle with 1 Tbsp toasted almonds.

Nutrition Tip:
This simple, delicious breakfast is a great source of calcium, which is needed for bone health and the prevention of osteoporosis.

Exchanges/Choices
1 Fat-Free Milk
1 Carbohydrate
1 Fat

Calories	195
Calories from Fat	40
Total Fat	4.5 g
Saturated Fat	0.6 g
Trans Fat	0 g
Cholesterol	15 mg
Sodium	160 mg
Total Carbohydrate	26 g
Dietary Fiber	1 g
Sugars	23 g
Protein	14 g

lunch

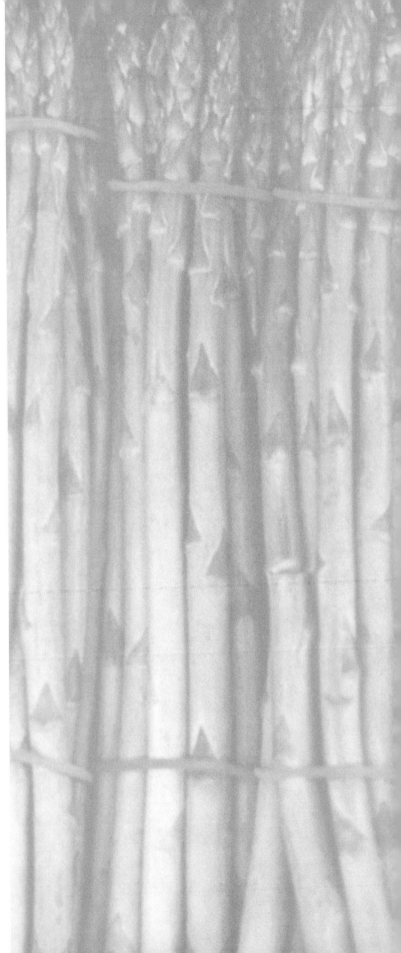

BALSAMIC AND FETA PIZZA

Serves 8 • Serving Size: 1 slice • Prep Time: 15 minutes

1/2 cup balsamic vinegar

1 (12-inch) prepackaged whole-wheat Italian pizza crust

Olive oil spray

2 garlic cloves, minced

2 plum (roma) tomatoes, sliced

1/3 cup reduced-fat feta cheese, crumbled

1. Preheat oven to 375°F.

2. Add balsamic vinegar to a small saucepan over medium-high heat. Bring to a boil. Reduce to a simmer and cook until vinegar becomes a syrup (about 10 minutes).

3. Lightly spray pizza crust with olive oil. Sprinkle minced garlic on top. Spread balsamic syrup evenly over crust. Arrange the tomato slices around the pizza.

4. Sprinkle the cheese on top and bake on rack in the oven for 10 minutes.

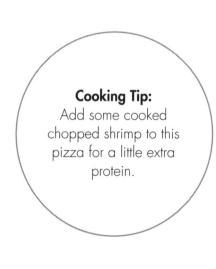

Cooking Tip:
Add some cooked chopped shrimp to this pizza for a little extra protein.

Exchanges/Choices
1 Starch
1 Vegetable
1/2 Fat

Calories	120
Calories from Fat	20
Total Fat	2.5 g
Saturated Fat	1.4 g
Trans Fat	0 g
Cholesterol	0 mg
Sodium	265 mg
Total Carbohydrate	21 g
Dietary Fiber	3 g
Sugars	4 g
Protein	6 g

BEET AND GOAT CHEESE SALAD WITH CHICKEN

Serves 5 • Serving Size: 1/5th recipe • Prep Time: 10 minutes

1 5-oz bag mixed baby field greens

1 15-oz can sliced beets, drained

1 4-oz boneless, skinless chicken breast, cooked and sliced

1 Tbsp goat cheese, crumbled

1/4 cup green onion, chopped

3 Tbsp red wine vinegar

1 Tbsp olive oil

1 tsp Splenda

1/2 tsp salt (*optional*)

1. In a medium bowl, add mixed baby field greens. Top with sliced beets, sliced chicken, and crumbled goat cheese.

2. In a small bowl whisk together green onions, vinegar, olive oil, Splenda, and salt (optional).

3. Drizzle dressing over salad.

Exchanges/Choices
1 Vegetable
1 Fat

Calories	80
Calories from Fat	35
Total Fat	4 g
Saturated Fat	0.9 g
Trans Fat	0 g
Cholesterol	15 mg
Sodium	130 mg
Total Carbohydrate	6 g
Dietary Fiber	1 g
Sugars	4 g
Protein	6 g

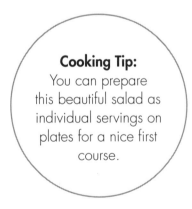

Cooking Tip:
You can prepare this beautiful salad as individual servings on plates for a nice first course.

BLACK BEAN BURGERS

Serves 8 • Serving Size: 1 burger • Prep Time: 15 minutes

2 15-oz cans black beans, rinsed and drained

3/4 cup salsa, divided

1 large egg

1/2 cup cornmeal

1 green bell pepper, finely diced

3 green onions, chopped

1 tsp chili powder

1/2 tsp cumin

1/4 tsp cayenne pepper

1/4 tsp ground black pepper

1/2 cup light sour cream

8 whole-wheat hamburger buns

Cooking Tip:
These burgers also make a great appetizer, just shape into smaller patties, take away the bun, and top with salsa and sour cream.

1. Puree 1 can black beans, 1/4 cup salsa, and egg in a blender or food processor until smooth.

2. In a large bowl, mix together pureed beans, remaining 1 can of black beans, cornmeal, green pepper, onions, chili powder, cumin, cayenne pepper, and pepper.

3. Form bean mixture into eight 1/2-inch thick patties.

4. Coat a large skillet with cooking spray and heat over medium heat. Add black bean burgers to skillet (working in batches), cook about 3 minutes per side, until they begin to brown. Serve black bean burgers on buns, topped with dollop of sour cream and salsa.

Exchanges/Choices
3 Starch
1/2 Fat

Calories 270	
Calories from Fat.....40	
Total Fat ....4.5 g	
Saturated Fat ....1.7 g	
Trans Fat ....0 g	
Cholesterol ....30 mg	
Sodium ....455 mg	
Total Carbohydrate ....47 g	
Dietary Fiber ....10 g	
Sugars ....7 g	
Protein ....12 g	

BLACK BEAN AND CHEESE QUESADILLA

Serves 6 • Serving Size: 1 quesadilla • Prep Time: Less than 5 minutes

Cooking spray

6 whole-wheat tortillas*

9 Tbsp reduced-fat, shredded, Mexican-style cheese

3/4 cup black bean and corn salsa

1/4 cup fat-free sour cream

1. Spray a large nonstick skillet with cooking spray and add one tortilla to pan.

2. Top tortilla with 1 1/2 Tbsp cheese and 2 Tbsp salsa and fold tortilla in half. Grill about 2 minutes on each side.

3. Top quesadilla with 2 tsp sour cream.

4. Repeat procedure for remaining five quesadillas.

Cooking Tip:
These quesadillas are great when served with a side salad topped with Southwest dressing; just mix together some salsa and light ranch dressing for a tasty twist.

Exchanges/Choices
2 Starch
1 Fat

Calories 220
  Calories from Fat.....55
Total Fat ....6 g
  Saturated Fat ....1.4 g
  Trans Fat ....0 g
Cholesterol ....10 mg
Sodium ....650 mg
Total Carbohydrate ....31 g
  Dietary Fiber ....5 g
  Sugars ....2 g
Protein ....8 g

Each tortilla should have 30 g carbohydrate and 4 g dietary fiber per serving.

This recipe is high in sodium.

BLT SALAD

Serves 6 • Serving Size: 1 1/2 cups • Prep Time: 20 minutes

3 slices whole-wheat bread, cut into 1/2-inch cubes

1 Tbsp olive oil

1/2 tsp garlic salt

Cooking spray

6 slices turkey bacon, cut into 1-inch pieces, cooked to crisp

3 tomatoes, cut into eighths

1 6-oz bag mixed lettuce

1/2 cup light ranch dressing

1. Preheat oven to 375°F.

2. Toss bread cubes in olive oil and garlic salt. Spray a baking sheet with cooking spray. Bake bread cubes on sheet for 15–20 minutes or until golden brown to make croutons. Set aside.

3. In a large bowl, toss all remaining ingredients. Top with warm croutons.

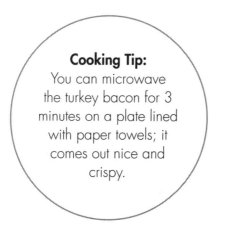

Cooking Tip:
You can microwave the turkey bacon for 3 minutes on a plate lined with paper towels; it comes out nice and crispy.

Exchanges/Choices
1/2 Starch
1 Vegetable
1 1/2 Fat

Calories	135
Calories from Fat	70
Total Fat	8 g
Saturated Fat	1.4 g
Trans Fat	0 g
Cholesterol	15 mg
Sodium	450 mg
Total Carbohydrate	11 g
Dietary Fiber	2 g
Sugars	4 g
Protein	5 g

BUFFALO CHICKEN PITA

Serves 4 • Serving Size: 1/2 pita pocket • Prep Time: 10 minutes

2 cups cooked and chopped chicken breast

1 cup celery, chopped

1/4 cup bottled buffalo wing sauce

4 romaine lettuce leaves

4 Tbsp reduced-fat bleu cheese salad dressing

2 whole-wheat pita pockets

1. In a large bowl, combine chicken, celery, and buffalo wing sauce. Stir to coat all chicken evenly.

2. Cut pitas in half to form pockets. Fill one half with one lettuce leaf, 1 Tbsp bleu cheese dressing, and 1/2 cup chicken salad mixture. Repeat for remaining three pita halves.

Exchanges/Choices
1 1/2 Starch
3 Lean Meat

Calories 250
   Calories from Fat.....55
Total Fat ....6 g
   Saturated Fat ....1.4 g
   Trans Fat ....0 g
Cholesterol ....60 mg
Sodium ....770 mg
Total Carbohydrate ....21 g
   Dietary Fiber ....3 g
   Sugars ....2 g
Protein.....................26 g

Nutrition Tip:
Look at the nutrition information on the bottle of buffalo wing sauce and find one that is the lowest in total carbohydrates and sodium.

CALIFORNIA TURKEY SANDWICH

Serves 4 • Serving Size: 1 sandwich • Prep Time: 5 minutes

3 Tbsp light mayonnaise

1 jalapeño pepper, seeded and minced

8 slices whole-wheat bread

1 avocado, sliced

12 oz oven-roasted turkey breast lunchmeat, sliced

8 romaine lettuce leaves

2 tomatoes, cut into 8 slices

1. In a blender or food processor, combine the mayonnaise and jalapeño pepper.

2. Spread mayonnaise evenly over four slices of whole-wheat bread.

3. Top each slice of bread with 1/4 avocado, 3 oz turkey lunchmeat, 2 romaine lettuce leaves, 2 tomato slices, and another slice of whole-wheat bread.

4. Repeat for remaining three sandwiches.

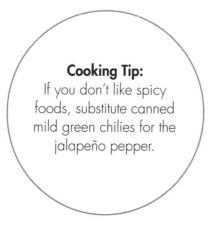

Cooking Tip:
If you don't like spicy foods, substitute canned mild green chilies for the jalapeño pepper.

Exchanges/Choices
2 Starch
1 Vegetable
4 Lean Meat
1 Fat

Calories 400
    Calories from Fat...135
Total Fat ....15 g
    Saturated Fat ....3.2 g
    Trans Fat ....0 g
Cholesterol ....70 mg
Sodium ....425 mg
Total Carbohydrate ....32 g
    Dietary Fiber ....8 g
    Sugars ....6 g
Protein ....34 g

the healthy carb diabetes cookbook

CAPRESE PANINI

Serves 8 • Serving Size: 1/2 sandwich • Prep Time: 5 minutes

2 medium tomatoes, thinly sliced into 8 slices
1/2 tsp garlic powder
8 whole basil leaves
3/4 cup reduced-fat, shredded mozzarella cheese
8 slices whole-wheat bread
Olive oil spray

1. Prepare an indoor or outdoor grill or panini maker.

2. Sprinkle tomato slices with garlic powder. Add two tomato slices, two basil leaves, and 3 Tbsp shredded cheese to one piece of bread. Top with another piece of bread and spray both sides of the sandwich with olive oil spray. Repeat for remaining three sandwiches.

3. Grill sandwiches on heated panini maker or on heated indoor or outdoor grill for 3–4 minutes on each side, pressing down as they grill.

Exchanges/Choices
1 Starch
1/2 Fat

Calories 105
 Calories from Fat 20
Total Fat .... 2.5 g
 Saturated Fat .... 1.2 g
 Trans Fat .... 0 g
Cholesterol .... 5 mg
Sodium .... 210 mg
Total Carbohydrate .... 13 g
 Dietary Fiber .... 2 g
 Sugars .... 3 g
Protein .... 7 g

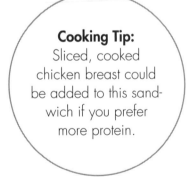

Cooking Tip:
Sliced, cooked chicken breast could be added to this sandwich if you prefer more protein.

CHICKEN PESTO PANINI

Serves 4 • Serving Size: 1 sandwich • Prep Time: 10 minutes

4 4-oz boneless, skinless chicken breasts
  (pounded thin)

1 Tbsp dried oregano

1/2 tsp ground black pepper

Cooking spray

4 Tbsp jarred pesto sauce

8 slices whole-wheat bread

4 tomato slices

4 tsp freshly grated Parmesan cheese

Cooking spray

Cooking Tip:
This sandwich can also be grilled in a heavy skillet coated with cooking spray. Press down on the sandwiches with another heavy pan and cook for 4 minutes on each side over medium-high heat.

1. Prepare an indoor grill or a panini maker.

2. Season chicken breasts with oregano and black pepper. Spray sauté pan with cooking spray and heat over medium heat. Add chicken breast and cook about 5 minutes each side or until done. Remove from heat.

3. To assemble sandwiches, spread 1 Tbsp pesto sauce on both sides of each cooked chicken breast, and then place one chicken breast on top of one slice of bread. Top with a tomato slice, 1 tsp of cheese, and another slice of bread. Repeat this process for the remaining three sandwiches.

4. Spray sandwiches with cooking spray and grill sandwiches on a heated panini maker or heated indoor grill for 5–7 minutes.

Exchanges/Choices
2 Starch
4 Lean Meat

Calories	325
Calories from Fat	90
Total Fat	10 g
Saturated Fat	2.3 g
Trans Fat	0 g
Cholesterol	70 mg
Sodium	515 mg
Total Carbohydrate	26 g
Dietary Fiber	5 g
Sugars	4 g
Protein	33 g

the healthy carb diabetes cookbook

CHICKEN SALAD WITH GRAPES AND WALNUTS

Serves 10 • Serving Size: 1/2 cup • Prep Time: 20 minutes

3 cups cooked chicken breast, chopped (about 2 medium breasts)

1 cup chopped celery (about 4 stalks)

2 cups seedless red grapes, sliced

1/4 cup walnuts, chopped

1/2 cup nonfat plain yogurt

1/2 cup light mayonnaise

1/4 tsp salt (*optional*)

1/4 tsp ground black pepper

1. In a large bowl, combine the chicken, celery, grapes, and walnuts. Gently stir to incorporate.

2. In a small bowl, whisk together the yogurt, mayonnaise, salt (optional), and pepper. Pour over chicken mixture and gently stir to coat.

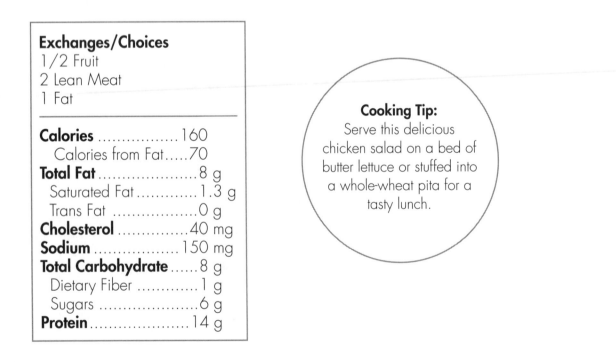

Exchanges/Choices
1/2 Fruit
2 Lean Meat
1 Fat

Calories 160
  Calories from Fat.....70
Total Fat .... 8 g
  Saturated Fat .... 1.3 g
  Trans Fat .... 0 g
Cholesterol .... 40 mg
Sodium .... 150 mg
Total Carbohydrate ...... 8 g
  Dietary Fiber .... 1 g
  Sugars .... 6 g
Protein .... 14 g

Cooking Tip:
Serve this delicious chicken salad on a bed of butter lettuce or stuffed into a whole-wheat pita for a tasty lunch.

CHINESE CHICKEN SALAD

Serves 6 • Serving Size: 1/6th recipe • Prep Time: 10 minutes

Salad

1 12-oz bag iceberg and romaine
lettuce with carrots

1/4 cup chopped green onions

1/4 cup roasted, salted peanuts,
chopped

2 cups cooked and chopped chicken
breast

1 11-oz can mandarin oranges in
juice, drained

Dressing

1/4 cup rice wine vinegar

1 Tbsp peanut butter

1 tsp hot sauce (optional)

1 Tbsp lite soy sauce

2 tsp sesame oil

2 Tbsp canola oil

1. In a large bowl, combine the lettuce, green onions, peanuts, cooked chicken,
and mandarin oranges; toss.

2. In a small bowl, whisk together the vinegar, peanut butter, hot sauce, soy
sauce, and sesame and canola oil.

3. Pour dressing over salad; toss to coat.

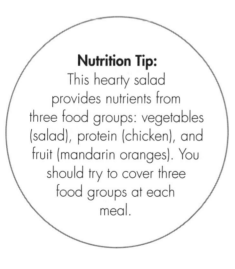

Nutrition Tip:
This hearty salad
provides nutrients from
three food groups: vegetables
(salad), protein (chicken), and
fruit (mandarin oranges). You
should try to cover three
food groups at each
meal.

Exchanges/Choices
1/2 Carbohydrate
1 Lean Meat
2 Fat

Calories 180
Calories from Fat...110
Total Fat ....12 g
Saturated Fat ....1.5 g
Trans Fat ....0 g
Cholesterol ....25 mg
Sodium ....190 mg
Total Carbohydrate ......8 g
Dietary Fiber ....2 g
Sugars ....5 g
Protein ....12 g

CRAB SALAD

Serves 4 • Serving Size: 1/2 cup • Prep Time: 5 minutes

2 6-oz cans lump white crabmeat, drained

1/2 green pepper, finely diced

1/4 cup light mayonnaise

1/4 cup nonfat plain yogurt

2 Tbsp fresh chives, chopped

1/4 tsp salt (*optional*)

1/8 tsp ground black pepper

4 large Bibb lettuce leaves

2 green onions, chopped

1. In a medium bowl, combine all ingredients except the green onions and Bibb lettuce.

2. Scoop 1/2 cup crab salad and place on top of one Bibb lettuce leaf. Top with green onions. Repeat for remaining three lettuce leaves.

Exchanges/Choices
2 Lean Meat
1/2 Fat

Calories 120
   Calories from Fat.....55
Total Fat ....6 g
   Saturated Fat ....1 g
   Trans Fat ....0 g
Cholesterol ....55 mg
Sodium ....335 mg
Total Carbohydrate ......4 g
   Dietary Fiber ....1 g
   Sugars ....2 g
Protein ....13 g

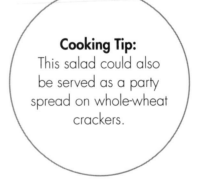

Cooking Tip:
This salad could also be served as a party spread on whole-wheat crackers.

CURRIED COUSCOUS WITH TURKEY

Serves 4 • Serving Size: 1 cup • Prep Time: 15 minutes

1/2 lb lean ground turkey breast

1/2 tsp cumin

1/2 tsp garlic powder

1/4 tsp cayenne pepper

1 1/2 cups reduced-sodium, fat-free chicken broth

1 tsp curry powder

1/2 tsp ground black pepper

3/4 cup whole-wheat couscous, uncooked

2 green onions, thinly sliced (white and green part)

1/4 cup Italian parsley, chopped

1. In a medium skillet, cook turkey over medium-high heat. Add cumin, garlic powder, and cayenne pepper. Cook until meat is brown.

2. In a small saucepan, boil chicken broth, curry powder, and black pepper. Add couscous; cover and remove from heat. Let sit for 5 minutes, then fluff with a fork.

3. Place couscous in a large bowl. Add cooked turkey, green onions, and parsley, and mix well. Serve warm.

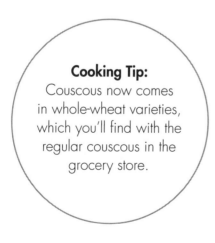

Cooking Tip:
Couscous now comes in whole-wheat varieties, which you'll find with the regular couscous in the grocery store.

Exchanges/Choices
1 1/2 Starch
2 Lean Meat

Calories	175
Calories from Fat	15
Total Fat	1.5 g
Saturated Fat	0.3 g
Trans Fat	0 g
Cholesterol	35 mg
Sodium	220 mg
Total Carbohydrate	23 g
Dietary Fiber	2 g
Sugars	1 g
Protein	19 g

CURRY CHICKEN WRAPS

Serves 6 • Serving Size: 1 wrap • Prep Time: 15 minutes

1 1/4 lb boneless, skinless chicken breasts, cooked and shredded

2 green onions, chopped

1 1/2 tsp curry powder

3 Tbsp light mayonnaise

2 Tbsp nonfat plain yogurt

2 Tbsp raisins

1/4 tsp ground black pepper

6 whole-wheat tortilla wraps*

1. In a medium bowl combine all ingredients except tortillas.

2. Scoop 1/2 cup chicken salad into tortilla wrap. Fold in the left and right sides of the tortilla, until the edges are about 1 inch apart, and then roll from the top down. Repeat entire process for remaining five wraps.

Exchanges/Choices
2 Starch
3 Lean Meat
1/2 Fat

Calories	310
Calories from Fat	70
Total Fat	8 g
Saturated Fat	1.3 g
Trans Fat	0 g
Cholesterol	55 mg
Sodium	505 mg
Total Carbohydrate	32 g
Dietary Fiber	5 g
Sugars	4 g
Protein	25 g

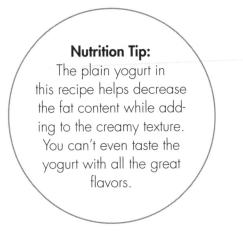

Nutrition Tip:
The plain yogurt in this recipe helps decrease the fat content while adding to the creamy texture. You can't even taste the yogurt with all the great flavors.

*Each tortilla should have 30 g carbohydrate and 4 g dietary fiber per serving.

FISH SANDWICH

Serves 4 • Serving Size: 1 sandwich • Prep Time: 5 minutes

Cooking spray

4 lemon pepper frozen fish fillets
   (not breaded)

4 whole-wheat hamburger buns

4 romaine lettuce leaves

4 tomato slices

Tartar Sauce

2 Tbsp light mayonnaise

1 tsp sweet pickle relish

1. Preheat oven to 350°F. Coat a baking sheet with cooking spray.

2. Bake fish fillets according to package directions.

3. In a small bowl, mix together ingredients for tartar sauce.

4. Spread 1 tsp tartar sauce on bottom side of hamburger bun. Top with fish fillet, lettuce leaf, tomato slice, and top of hamburger bun. Repeat for remaining three sandwiches.

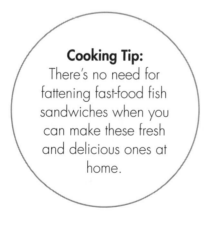

Cooking Tip:
There's no need for fattening fast-food fish sandwiches when you can make these fresh and delicious ones at home.

Exchanges/Choices
1 1/2 Starch
3 Lean Meat

Calories	240
Calories from Fat	45
Total Fat	5 g
Saturated Fat	0.9 g
Trans Fat	0 g
Cholesterol	50 mg
Sodium	525 mg
Total Carbohydrate	25 g
Dietary Fiber	4 g
Sugars	5 g
Protein	24 g

the healthy carb diabetes cookbook

FIVE BEAN SOUP

Serves 15 • Serving Size: 1 cup • Prep Time: 5 minutes

Cooking spray

14 oz lean smoked turkey sausage (kielbasa), sliced

1 cup diced celery

1 medium onion, diced

1 carrot, diced

1 15.5-oz can kidney beans, rinsed and drained

1 15.5-oz can pinto beans, rinsed and drained

1 15.5-oz can navy beans, rinsed and drained

1 15.5-oz can black beans, rinsed and drained

1 15.5-oz can black eyed peas, rinsed and drained

2 32-oz cans reduced-sodium, fat-free chicken broth

1 14.5-oz can no-salt-added diced tomato

1 Tbsp dried basil

1 Tbsp dried oregano

1/4 tsp cayenne pepper (*optional*)

1/2 tsp salt (*optional*)

1 tsp ground black pepper

1 bay leaf

1. Coat a large soup pot with cooking spray. Over medium-high heat, sauté sausage until lightly browned. Remove from pan.

2. Add celery, onion, and carrot to pot and sauté over medium-high heat for approximately 4 minutes.

3. Return the sausage to the pot and add all remaining ingredients. Bring to a boil; reduce heat and simmer for 25 minutes.

4. Remove bay leaf and serve.

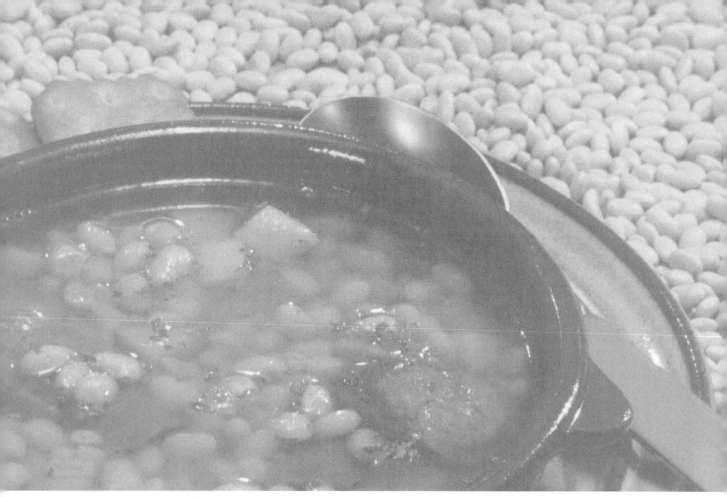

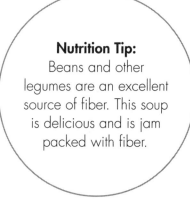

Nutrition Tip:
Beans and other legumes are an excellent source of fiber. This soup is delicious and is jam packed with fiber.

This recipe is high in sodium.

Exchanges/Choices
1 1/2 Starch
1 Vegetable
1 Lean Meat

Calories 180
   Calories from Fat 20
Total Fat .... 2 g
   Saturated Fat .... 0.5 g
   Trans Fat .... 0 g
Cholesterol .... 15 mg
Sodium .... 705 mg
Total Carbohydrate .... 27 g
   Dietary Fiber .... 8 g
   Sugars .... 4 g
Protein .... 14 g

GAZPACHO

Serves 6 • Serving Size: 1/6th recipe • Prep Time: 25 minutes

4 medium ripe tomatoes, chopped

3 cloves garlic, minced

2 cucumbers, peeled, seeded, and chopped

2 celery stalks, chopped

1 medium red onion, chopped

1 green bell pepper, cored, seeded, and chopped

4 cups no-salt-added tomato juice

1/4 cup red wine (can substitute 2 Tbsp balsamic vinegar)

2 Tbsp olive oil

2 Tbsp hot sauce (*optional*)

1/4 tsp salt (*optional*)

1/2 tsp ground black pepper

1. Place all ingredients in a large bowl and mix well; reserve 2 cups. Working in batches, blend the mixture in a blender or food processor until just slightly chunky. Stir in reserved 2 cups.

2. Serve chilled.

Exchanges/Choices
3 Vegetable
1 Fat

Calories	120
Calories from Fat	45
Total Fat	5 g
Saturated Fat	0.7 g
Trans Fat	0 g
Cholesterol	0 mg
Sodium	40 mg
Total Carbohydrate	17 g
Dietary Fiber	3 g
Sugars	11 g
Protein	3 g

Cooking Tip:
This cold soup is served best on a hot summer's day, when all of this produce is at its peak season.

GREEK CHICKEN SALAD

Serves 5 • Serving Size: 1/5th recipe • Prep Time: 5 minutes

Salad

15 oz romaine lettuce, cut into pieces

10 oz precooked, packaged chicken
(about 2 cups)

10 kalamata olives, pitted

3 oz reduced-fat feta cheese,
crumbled

Dressing

2 Tbsp lemon juice

1 Tbsp olive oil

1/2 tsp dried oregano

1/4 tsp ground black pepper

1 tsp Splenda

1. In a large bowl, mix together all salad ingredients. In a small bowl, whisk together dressing ingredients.

2. Pour dressing over salad and toss to coat.

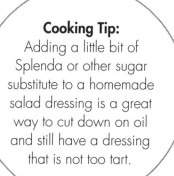

Cooking Tip:
Adding a little bit of Splenda or other sugar substitute to a homemade salad dressing is a great way to cut down on oil and still have a dressing that is not too tart.

Exchanges/Choices
1 Vegetable
2 Lean Meat
1/2 Fat

Calories 145
Calories from Fat 65
Total Fat .... 7 g
Saturated Fat .... 2 g
Trans Fat .... 0 g
Cholesterol .... 35 mg
Sodium .... 465 mg
Total Carbohydrate ...... 4 g
Dietary Fiber .... 2 g
Sugars .... 1 g
Protein .... 18 g

GREEN ITALIAN TUNA SALAD

Serves 4 • Serving Size: 2 cups • Prep Time: 10 minutes

Salad

1 10-oz bag Italian-style lettuce

2 plum (roma) tomatoes, diced

2 Tbsp sliced black olives

2 3-oz pkg tuna packed in water, drained

2 Tbsp grated Parmesan cheese

Dressing

1 lemon, juiced

2 Tbsp olive oil

1 Tbsp balsamic vinegar

1/2 tsp dried basil

1/2 tsp dried oregano

1/4 tsp ground black pepper

1. In a large bowl, toss together salad ingredients.

2. In a small bowl, whisk together dressing ingredients.

3. Pour dressing over salad and toss to coat.

Exchanges/Choices
1 Vegetable
1 Lean Meat
1 1/2 Fat

Calories 150
   Calories from Fat..... 80
Total Fat .... 9 g
   Saturated Fat .... 1.6 g
   Trans Fat .... 0 g
Cholesterol .... 15 mg
Sodium .... 205 mg
Total Carbohydrate ...... 7 g
   Dietary Fiber .... 2 g
   Sugars .... 3 g
Protein .... 12 g

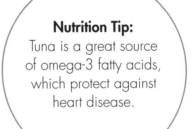

Nutrition Tip:
Tuna is a great source
of omega-3 fatty acids,
which protect against
heart disease.

HEALTHY TUNA

Serves 8 • Serving Size: 1/8th recipe • Prep Time: 10 minutes

3/4 cup shredded carrots (3 medium carrots)

2 medium celery stalks, diced

1/2 medium onion, shredded

4 hard-boiled egg whites, chopped

12 oz chunk white tuna packed in water, drained

1/4 cup nonfat plain yogurt

1/4 cup light mayonnaise

1/4 tsp salt (*optional*)

1/4 tsp ground black pepper

2 Tbsp Italian (flat leaf) parsley, chopped

1. In a medium bowl, combine all ingredients.

2. Serve tuna salad on whole-wheat toast, pita, or crackers.

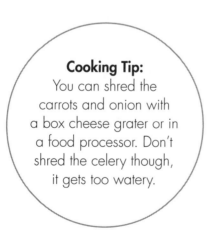

Cooking Tip:
You can shred the carrots and onion with a box cheese grater or in a food processor. Don't shred the celery though, it gets too watery.

Exchanges/Choices
2 Lean Meat

Calories 90
  Calories from Fat.....25
Total Fat ....3 g
  Saturated Fat............0.5 g
  Trans Fat ....0 g
Cholesterol ....15 mg
Sodium ....245 mg
Total Carbohydrate ......4 g
  Dietary Fiber ....1 g
  Sugars ....2 g
Protein ....12 g

the healthy carb diabetes cookbook

HEALTHY TURKEY BAGEL SANDWICH

Serves 4 • Serving Size: 1 sandwich • Prep Time: 5 minutes

4 tsp honey mustard

4 small whole-wheat bagels, toasted

8 oz thinly sliced, oven-roasted deli turkey

4 tsp sunflower seeds

1/2 cucumber, thinly sliced

4 romaine lettuce leaves

4 tomato slices

1. Spread 1 tsp mustard on one side of bagel. Add 2 oz turkey meat. Top with 1 tsp sunflower seeds, 4 cucumber slices, 1 romaine lettuce leaf, and 1 tomato slice.

2. Repeat procedure for remaining three sandwiches.

Exchanges/Choices
2 Starch
2 Lean Meat

Calories	240
Calories from Fat	35
Total Fat	4 g
Saturated Fat	0.9 g
Trans Fat	0 g
Cholesterol	25 mg
Sodium	765 mg
Total Carbohydrate	34 g
Dietary Fiber	5 g
Sugars	7 g
Protein	21 g

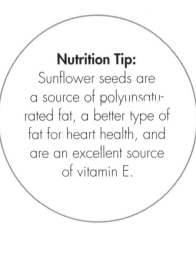

Nutrition Tip:
Sunflower seeds are a source of polyunsaturated fat, a better type of fat for heart health, and are an excellent source of vitamin E.

This recipe is high in sodium.

HOT HAM AND SWISS SANDWICH

Serves 4 • Serving Size: 1 sandwich • Prep Time: 10 minutes

4 tsp honey Dijon mustard

8 slices whole-wheat bread

4 (3/4-oz) wedges light Swiss cheese (Laughing Cow brand)

8 oz deli-style ham

1 medium tomato, sliced

8 slices red onion

Cooking spray

1. Prepare an indoor grill or a panini maker.

2. Spread 1 tsp Dijon mustard on 1 slice of bread. Spread 1 wedge of cheese on bread; top with 2 oz ham, 1 slice tomato, 2 onion slices, and the other slice of bread.

3. Spray the outside of the sandwiches with cooking spray. Repeat procedure for remaining three sandwiches.

4. Place sandwiches on heated indoor grill or panini maker and cook for 4–5 minutes, until bread is toasted and cheese is melted.

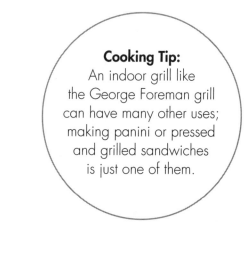

Cooking Tip:
An indoor grill like the George Foreman grill can have many other uses; making panini or pressed and grilled sandwiches is just one of them.

This recipe is high in sodium.

Exchanges/Choices
2 Starch
2 Lean Meat

Calories	250
Calories from Fat	55
Total Fat	6 g
Saturated Fat	2.5 g
Trans Fat	0 g
Cholesterol	40 mg
Sodium	1235 mg
Total Carbohydrate	30 g
Dietary Fiber	5 g
Sugars	7 g
Protein	19 g

MANGO SALSA SHRIMP

Serves 4 • Serving Size: 1/4th recipe • Prep Time: 10 minutes

1 tsp olive oil

1 Tbsp lime juice

1 mango, diced small (1 cup)

1/2 cup red onion, diced small

1 jalapeño pepper, seeded and minced

1 lb cooked shrimp, peeled and deveined

4 Bibb lettuce leaves

2 Tbsp chopped fresh cilantro

1. In a small bowl, whisk together the olive oil and lime juice. Add mango, red onion, jalapeño, and shrimp; toss to coat.

2. Fill each lettuce leaf with 1/4th of the shrimp-mango mixture. Garnish with chopped cilantro.

Exchanges/Choices
1/2 Fruit
2 Lean Meat

Calories 120
 Calories from Fat.....20
Total Fat .... 2 g
 Saturated Fat .... 0.4 g
 Trans Fat .... 0 g
Cholesterol .... 130 mg
Sodium .... 155 mg
Total Carbohydrate .... 11 g
 Dietary Fiber .... 1 g
 Sugars .... 8 g
Protein .... 15 g

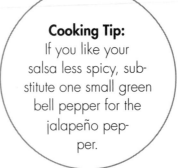

Cooking Tip:
If you like your salsa less spicy, substitute one small green bell pepper for the jalapeño pepper.

MEDITERRANEAN TUNA MELT

Serves 5 • Serving Size: 1 tuna melt • Prep Time: 5 minutes

2 6-oz cans tuna packed in water, drained

1/4 cup light mayonnaise

1/4 tsp ground black pepper

1/4 tsp onion powder

1 Tbsp lemon juice

3 Tbsp sun-dried tomatoes, chopped

5 whole-wheat English muffin halves

5 1-oz slices reduced-fat provolone cheese

1. Preheat oven to 400°F. In a medium mixing bowl, combine the tuna, mayonnaise, pepper, onion powder, lemon juice, and sun-dried tomatoes.

2. Spread 1/4 cup tuna mixture on top of each muffin half and top with 1 slice of cheese.

3. Place muffins on baking sheet and bake 10 minutes.

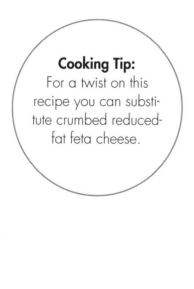

Cooking Tip:
For a twist on this recipe you can substitute crumbed reduced-fat feta cheese.

This recipe is high in sodium.

Exchanges/Choices	
1 Starch	
2 Lean Meat	
1/2 Fat	

Calories	200
Calories from Fat	55
Total Fat	6 g
Saturated Fat	1.5 g
Trans Fat	0 g
Cholesterol	25 mg
Sodium	505 mg
Total Carbohydrate	16 g
Dietary Fiber	3 g
Sugars	4 g
Protein	20 g

MEXICAN TUNA SALAD

Serves 6 • Serving Size: 1/2 pita pocket • Prep Time: 15 minutes

1 12-oz flavor-fresh tuna pouch, in water

1/4 cup light mayonnaise

3 Tbsp nonfat plain yogurt

1/4 cup onion, finely diced

1 large tomato, seeded and finely diced

1 jalapeño pepper, seeded and diced

1/3 cup fresh cilantro, chopped

1/4 tsp ground black pepper

6 whole-wheat pita pocket halves

1. In a medium mixing bowl, combine all ingredients except pita pocket halves.

2. Fill each pocket half with 1/6 of tuna mixture. Repeat process for remaining five pockets.

Exchanges/Choices
1 Starch
1 Vegetable
2 Lean Meat

Calories 195
   Calories from Fat..... 40
Total Fat .... 4.5 g
   Saturated Fat .... 0.8 g
   Trans Fat .... 0 g
Cholesterol .... 20 mg
Sodium .... 435 mg
Total Carbohydrate .... 22 g
   Dietary Fiber .... 3 g
   Sugars .... 3 g
Protein .... 17 g

Cooking Tip:
Whole-wheat pita pockets should be available at your local grocery store. If you are having trouble finding them, ask your grocer to order them.

NACHOS SUPREME

Serves 6 • Serving Size: 1/6th recipe • Prep Time: 10 minutes

6 oz whole-grain tortilla chips

1 1/2 cups fat-free refried beans, warmed

2 Tbsp pickled jalapeño slices (*see tip below*)

1/2 cup reduced-fat, shredded Mexican-style cheese

1/2 cup fat-free sour cream

1 tomato, seeded and diced

1 cup shredded lettuce

1. Preheat oven to 400°F.

2. Spread half the chips in a shallow casserole dish. Top with half the beans, in small spoonfuls, and scatter with half the jalapeños. Repeat with the remaining chips, beans, and jalapeños. Sprinkle the top of the nachos with the cheese.

3. Bake until heated through and the cheese melts, about 3–5 minutes.

4. Top the nachos with sour cream, tomatoes, and shredded lettuce.

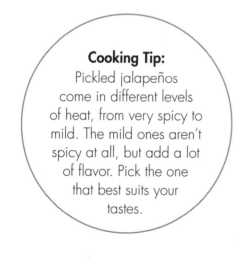

Cooking Tip:
Pickled jalapeños come in different levels of heat, from very spicy to mild. The mild ones aren't spicy at all, but add a lot of flavor. Pick the one that best suits your tastes.

Exchanges/Choices
2 Starch
1 Lean Meat
1 Fat

Calories	250
Calories from Fat	90
Total Fat	10 g
Saturated Fat	2.4 g
Trans Fat	0 g
Cholesterol	10 mg
Sodium	480 mg
Total Carbohydrate	29 g
Dietary Fiber	6 g
Sugars	3 g
Protein	9 g

QUICK CHICKEN SOUP

Serves 6 • Serving Size: 1 cup • Prep Time: 12 minutes

2 tsp trans-fat-free margarine

1 cup carrots, diced small

1 cup onions, diced small

1/2 cup celery, diced small

3 14.5-oz cans reduced-sodium, fat-free chicken broth

1 Tbsp parsley, chopped

1 bay leaf

1/4 cup instant brown rice

1/4 tsp ground black pepper

1 store-bought rotisserie whole cooked chicken (about 2 1/2 lb), skin removed and meat shredded

1. Heat margarine in a large soup pot over medium-high heat. Add carrots, onions, and celery, and sauté until the vegetables just begin to brown.

2. Add chicken broth (make sure to scrape off the brown bits on the bottom of the pan).

3. Add parsley, bay leaf, and rice; bring to a boil.

4. Reduce heat to a simmer; cover and cook for 10 minutes. Add pepper and shredded chicken. Cook for an additional 5 minutes. Remove bay leaf.

Exchanges/Choices
1/2 Starch
1 Vegetable
3 Lean Meat

Calories 190
   Calories from Fat 55
Total Fat .... 6 g
   Saturated Fat .... 1.6 g
   Trans Fat .... 0 g
Cholesterol .... 55 mg
Sodium .... 590 mg
Total Carbohydrate .... 12 g
   Dietary Fiber .... 2 g
   Sugars .... 3 g
Protein .... 21 g

Cooking Tip:
Store-bought cooked rotisserie chickens are delicious and can be a great time saver in the kitchen. They are usually found in the deli section of your grocery store.

ROAST BEEF SANDWICH

Serves 4 • Serving Size: 1 sandwich • Prep Time: 5 minutes

8 tsp light vegetable cream cheese

8 slices whole-wheat bread

8 oz deli-style lean roast beef, thinly sliced

4 romaine lettuce leaves

4 tomato slices

1. Spread 2 tsp cream cheese on 1 slice of bread. Top each sandwich with 2 oz roast beef, 1 lettuce leaf, 1 tomato slice, and 1 slice of bread.

2. Repeat this procedure for remaining three sandwiches.

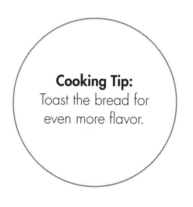

Cooking Tip:
Toast the bread for
even more flavor.

Exchanges/Choices
2 Starch
2 Lean Meat
1/2 Fat

Calories 255
   Calories from Fat.....55
Total Fat ....6 g
   Saturated Fat ....2.3 g
   Trans Fat ....0 g
Cholesterol ....40 mg
Sodium ....590 mg
Total Carbohydrate ....25 g
   Dietary Fiber ....4 g
   Sugars ....5 g
Protein ....24 g

SHRIMP LETTUCE WRAPS

Serves 6 • Serving Size: 1 wrap • Prep Time: 10 minutes

Sauce

3 green onions, minced

1 clove garlic, minced

1 pinch crushed red pepper flakes

1 Tbsp lite soy sauce

1/4 cup rice wine vinegar

1 Tbsp sesame oil

1 Tbsp Splenda

Shrimp

Cooking spray

1 lb raw shrimp, peeled and deveined

6 Bibb lettuce leaves

1 1/2 cups carrots, shredded

1 1/2 cups canned bean sprouts, rinsed and drained

2 Tbsp chopped fresh cilantro

1. In a large bowl, whisk together sauce ingredients.

2. Coat a medium nonstick skillet over medium heat with cooking spray. Add shrimp and sauté for 2 minutes. Remove shrimp from pan and add sauce. Cook sauce until it is reduced to a syrupy consistency, about 4–5 minutes. Return shrimp into sauce and sauté for 2 more minutes.

3. Divide shrimp evenly among the lettuce leaves and place in center of leaf. Top each lettuce leaf with 1/4 cup carrots, 1/4 cup bean sprouts, and 1 tsp cilantro.

Cooking Tip:
You can serve these wraps unassembled on a large tray and let your guests assemble their own for a fun and refreshing meal.

Exchanges/Choices
1 Vegetable
1 Lean Meat
1/2 Fat

Calories	90
Calories from Fat	25
Total Fat	3 g
Saturated Fat	0.5 g
Trans Fat	0 g
Cholesterol	85 mg
Sodium	230 mg
Total Carbohydrate	6 g
Dietary Fiber	2 g
Sugars	3 g
Protein	11 g

SPINACH FRITTATA

Serves 8 • Serving Size: 1 slice • Prep Time: 10 minutes

1 Tbsp olive oil

1 small onion, sliced into thin 1-inch strips

4 oz fresh spinach

2 whole eggs

3 egg whites

1/2 tsp salt (*optional*)

1/4 tsp ground black pepper

1/4 cup shredded reduced-fat cheddar cheese

1. Preheat broiler.

2. Add oil to a medium-sized, oven-safe sauté pan over medium heat. Add onions and sauté until tender, about 3–4 minutes. Add spinach and sauté until wilted, about 3–4 more minutes.

3. In a medium bowl, whisk together eggs, egg whites, salt (optional), and pepper. Pour egg mixture over the onions and spinach. Reduce heat to medium-low and let egg begin to set. Sprinkle cheese evenly over frittata.

4. Place frittata under the broiler for 2–3 minutes to melt cheese and cook the top of the frittata. Slide out of pan and cut into eight slices.

Cooking Tip:
When you're making meals that start on top of the stove and are finished in the oven or broiler, oven-safe sauté pans can save you from washing a lot of dishes later because you just use one pan.

Exchanges/Choices
1 Lean Meat
1/2 Fat

Calories	60
Calories from Fat	35
Total Fat	4 g
Saturated Fat	1.1 g
Trans Fat	0 g
Cholesterol	55 mg
Sodium	80 mg
Total Carbohydrate	2 g
Dietary Fiber	1 g
Sugars	1 g
Protein	4 g

THAI CHICKEN WRAP

Serves 5 • Serving Size: 1 wrap • Prep Time: 15 minutes

2 Tbsp creamy peanut butter (heated in microwave for 10 seconds)

1 Tbsp sugar-free apricot jelly

1 tsp lite soy sauce

2 Tbsp rice wine vinegar

1/4 tsp crushed red pepper flakes

2 green onions, chopped

1 cup shredded carrots

1/4 cup chopped fresh cilantro

2 4-oz boneless, skinless chicken breasts, cooked and chopped

5 whole-wheat tortillas*

1. In a medium bowl, whisk together peanut butter, jelly, soy sauce, vinegar, and red pepper flakes. Add remaining ingredients except tortillas, and toss to coat.

2. Fill each tortilla with 1/2 cup chicken mixture. Fold in left and right sides of tortillas until they touch and roll from the top down to make the wrap.

Exchanges/Choices
2 Starch
1 Vegetable
1 Lean Meat
1 Fat

Calories 275
    Calories from Fat.....70
Total Fat....................8 g
    Saturated Fat............1.2 g
    Trans Fat ....0 g
Cholesterol ....25 mg
Sodium ....505 mg
Total Carbohydrate....33 g
    Dietary Fiber ....6 g
    Sugars ....4 g
Protein....................16 g

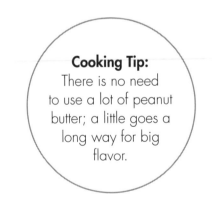

Cooking Tip:
There is no need
to use a lot of peanut
butter; a little goes a
long way for big
flavor.

Each tortilla should have 30 g carbohydrate and 4 g dietary fiber per serving.

TOMATO BASIL BISQUE

Serves 8 • Serving Size: 1/8th recipe • Prep Time: 10 minutes

1 Tbsp olive oil

1 medium onion, diced

1 cup celery, chopped

1 clove garlic, minced

2 28-oz cans no-salt-added crushed tomatoes

1 cup reduced-sodium, fat-free chicken broth

1/2 cup fresh basil, chopped

1 1/2 cups fat-free half-and-half

1 tsp salt (*optional*)

1/2 tsp ground black pepper

1. Add oil to a large soup pot over medium-high heat. Add onion and celery; sauté for 5–6 minutes or until onions turn clear.

2. Add garlic and sauté 1 minute. Add tomatoes and chicken broth and bring to a boil. Reduce to a simmer for 15 minutes, stirring occasionally.

3. Add basil and simmer 5 more minutes. Remove from heat and stir in half-and-half, salt (optional), and ground black pepper.

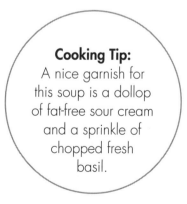

Cooking Tip:
A nice garnish for this soup is a dollop of fat-free sour cream and a sprinkle of chopped fresh basil.

Exchanges/Choices
1/2 Fat-Free Milk
2 Vegetable

Calories	95
Calories from Fat	25
Total Fat	3 g
Saturated Fat	0.6 g
Trans Fat	0 g
Cholesterol	0 mg
Sodium	155 mg
Total Carbohydrate	15 g
Dietary Fiber	3 g
Sugars	8 g
Protein	4 g

the healthy carb diabetes cookbook

TUNA AND VEGGIE PASTA SALAD

Serves 5 • Serving Size: 2 cups • Prep Time: 5 minutes

2 cups whole-wheat elbow macaroni noodles, uncooked

1 cup broccoli florets

1 cup celery, chopped

1 cup grape tomatoes, cut in half

1/2 cup fat-free sour cream

1/4 cup light mayonnaise

1 12-oz can tuna packed in water, drained

1/4 tsp salt (*optional*)

1/4 tsp ground black pepper

1. Cook pasta according to package directions, omitting salt. Drain and rinse under cold water. Set aside.

2. In a salad bowl, combine cooked pasta with remaining ingredients; toss well. Refrigerate until serving.

Exchanges/Choices
2 Starch
1 Vegetable
2 Lean Meat

Calories 285
    Calories from Fat.....45
Total Fat ....5 g
    Saturated Fat ....0.9 g
    Trans Fat ....0 g
Cholesterol ....25 mg
Sodium ....345 mg
Total Carbohydrate ....36 g
    Dietary Fiber ....5 g
    Sugars ....4 g
Protein...................24 g

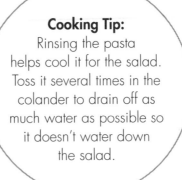

Cooking Tip:
Rinsing the pasta
helps cool it for the salad.
Toss it several times in the
colander to drain off as
much water as possible so
it doesn't water down
the salad.

TURKEY APPLE WRAP

Serves 4 • Serving Size: 1 wrap • Prep Time: 15 minutes

4 tsp honey mustard

4 whole-wheat tortillas*

12 oz low-sodium deli-style turkey breast, thinly sliced

1 gala apple, cored and diced with skin

2 oz sliced reduced-fat Swiss cheese

1. Spread 1 tsp mustard on one tortilla. Top tortilla with 3 oz turkey breast, 1/4 of diced apples, and 1/2 oz cheese. Fold left and right sides of tortilla in until they touch and roll from the top down to make the wrap.

2. Repeat procedure for remaining three wraps.

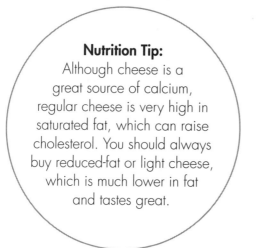

Nutrition Tip:
Although cheese is a great source of calcium, regular cheese is very high in saturated fat, which can raise cholesterol. You should always buy reduced-fat or light cheese, which is much lower in fat and tastes great.

Exchanges/Choices
2 Starch
4 Lean Meat

Calories	330
Calories from Fat	55
Total Fat	6 g
Saturated Fat	1.5 g
Trans Fat	0 g
Cholesterol	60 mg
Sodium	860 mg
Total Carbohydrate	34 g
Dietary Fiber	5 g
Sugars	6 g
Protein	29 g

*Each tortilla should have 30 g carbohydrate and 4 g dietary fiber per serving.

This recipe is high in sodium.

TURKEY ARTICHOKE WRAPS

Serves 6 • Serving Size: 1 wrap • Prep Time: 15 minutes

6 Tbsp light cream cheese with chives and onions

6 whole-wheat tortillas*

12 oz smoked deli-style turkey breast lunchmeat

1 14-oz can quartered artichoke hearts, drained

3 plum tomatoes, thinly sliced

1. Spread 1 Tbsp cream cheese on 1 tortilla. Add 2 oz turkey meat, 2 oz artichoke hearts, and 3 tomato slices.

2. Fold in the left and right side of the tortilla until the edges are about 1 inch apart and then roll from the top down. Repeat entire process for remaining five wraps.

Nutrition Tip:
If you like, mix up this recipe by trying any of the available flavored low-carb tortillas, such as spinach.

Exchanges/Choices
2 Starch
1 Vegetable
1 Lean Meat
1 Fat

Calories 270
   Calories from Fat.....65
Total Fat....................7 g
   Saturated Fat.............1.8 g
   Trans Fat ....0 g
Cholesterol..............25 mg
Sodium ....1005 mg
Total Carbohydrate....35 g
   Dietary Fiber ....5 g
   Sugars ....4 g
Protein....................16 g

Each tortilla should have 30 g carbohydrate and 4 g dietary fiber per serving.

This recipe is high in sodium.

TURKEY COBB SALAD

Serves 4 • Serving Size: 1 salad • Prep Time: 20 minutes

9 cups romaine lettuce, shredded

1 small cucumber, peeled and sliced into rounds

1 large tomato, quartered

1/2 avocado, quartered

8 oz oven-roasted turkey lunchmeat, cut into bite-sized pieces

2 hard boiled egg whites, cut in half

4 slices turkey bacon, cooked and chopped into 1-inch pieces

1/3 cup reduced-fat, shredded cheddar cheese

1/2 cup lite ranch dressing

1. Divide lettuce evenly on four plates (2 1/4 cups on each). Top each plate with two cucumber slices, one tomato wedge, one avocado wedge, 2 oz turkey, and one egg half. Evenly divide turkey bacon and cheddar cheese among four plates.

2. Top each salad with 2 Tbsp ranch dressing.

Exchanges/Choices
1/2 Carbohydrate
1 Vegetable
2 Lean Meat
2 1/2 Fat

Calories	255
Calories from Fat	135
Total Fat	15 g
Saturated Fat	3.1 g
Trans Fat	0 g
Cholesterol	41 mg
Sodium	1265 mg
Total Carbohydrate	11 g
Dietary Fiber	4 g
Sugars	5 g
Protein	21 g

Cooking Tip:
This recipe could also be made with chopped cooked chicken breast in place of the turkey.

This recipe is high in sodium.

TURKEY FLORENTINE SOUP

Serves 9 • Serving Size: 1 cup • Prep Time: 10 minutes

1 Tbsp olive oil

8 oz turkey breast, cooked and chopped

1 10-oz pkg chopped frozen spinach, thawed and drained

1 14.5-oz can no-salt-added diced tomatoes

1 garlic clove, minced

3 14.5-oz cans reduced-sodium, fat-free chicken broth, plus 1 can of water

1/2 tsp salt (*optional*)

1/2 tsp ground black pepper

1 cup whole-wheat elbow macaroni, uncooked

1. Heat olive oil in a medium soup pot over medium-high heat.

2. Add turkey, spinach, and tomatoes and sauté for 3–4 minutes. Add garlic and sauté 1 minute.

3. Add chicken broth, water, salt (optional), and pepper and bring to a boil.

4. Add the macaroni and reduce heat to a simmer for 10 minutes.

Exchanges/Choices
1/2 Starch
1 Vegetable
1 Lean Meat

Calories	110
Calories from Fat	20
Total Fat	2 g
Saturated Fat	0.3 g
Trans Fat	0 g
Cholesterol	15 mg
Sodium	390 mg
Total Carbohydrate	13 g
Dietary Fiber	3 g
Sugars	2 g
Protein	11 g

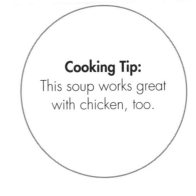

Cooking Tip:
This soup works great with chicken, too.

TURKEY GYROS

Serves 5 • Serving Size: 1 gyro • Prep Time: 15 minutes

1/4 cup lemon juice

1 tsp dried oregano

1 lb boneless, skinless turkey breasts, thinly sliced into strips

Cooking spray

1/4 tsp salt (*optional*)

1/4 tsp ground black pepper

4 whole-wheat pocket pitas

1 cup tomato, seeded and diced

5 Tbsp reduced-fat feta cheese, crumbled

Sauce

1 cup fat-free plain yogurt

1 cup cucumber, peeled and grated

1 clove garlic, minced

Nutrition Tip:
Fat-free yogurt is a good source of calcium. It's not just for breakfast anymore!

1. In a medium bowl, combine lemon juice and oregano, add turkey, and marinate in the refrigerator for 15 minutes.

2. Remove the turkey from the marinade and reserve 1 Tbsp of the marinade.

3. Coat a large nonstick sauté pan with cooking spray and heat over medium-high heat. Add turkey strips and reserved marinade to pan and sauté for 4–5 minutes or until the turkey is done. Add salt (optional) and pepper.

4. In a medium bowl, combine all sauce ingredients.

5. Fill each pita with 1 cup turkey, tomatoes, 1 Tbsp cheese, and 3 Tbsp sauce.

Exchanges/Choices
2 Starch
3 Lean Meat

Calories	270
Calories from Fat	25
Total Fat	3 g
Saturated Fat	1.2 g
Trans Fat	0 g
Cholesterol	65 mg
Sodium	430 mg
Total Carbohydrate	32 g
Dietary Fiber	4 g
Sugars	5 g
Protein	31 g

dinner

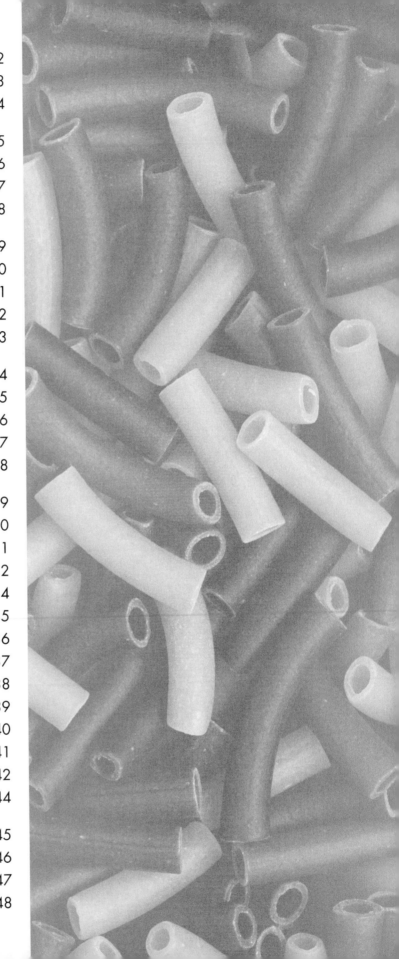

APRICOT-GLAZED PORK TENDERLOIN

Serves 8 • Serving Size: 1/8th recipe • Prep Time: 15 minutes

Cooking spray
2 lb pork tenderloin
3/4 tsp garlic powder
1 tsp cumin
1/2 tsp ground red pepper (*optional*)
1/2 tsp ground black pepper
1/2 tsp salt (*optional*)

Apricot Glaze
1/2 cup sugar-free apricot preserves
2 Tbsp apple cider

1. Preheat oven to 375°F. Spray a baking sheet with cooking spray.

2. Season the tenderloin well with garlic powder, cumin, red pepper, pepper, and salt (optional).

3. In a small saucepan over medium heat, add apricot preserves and cider; simmer for 3–5 minutes to form a glaze. Brush 1/4 cup apricot glaze on both sides of the tenderloin and transfer to a baking sheet. Bake for 40–50 minutes. Brush remaining apricot preserves evenly over pork and bake for an additional 10 minutes or until done.

4. Let pork sit for 10 minutes, slice thinly, and serve.

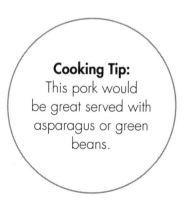

Cooking Tip:
This pork would be great served with asparagus or green beans.

Exchanges/Choices
3 Lean Meat

Calories 130
   Calories from Fat......25
Total Fat ....3 g
   Saturated Fat ....1 g
   Trans Fat ....0 g
Cholesterol ....60 mg
Sodium ....40 mg
Total Carbohydrate......3 g
   Dietary Fiber ....0 g
   Sugars ....0 g
Protein....................22 g

ASIAN BEEF KABOBS WITH BROWN RICE

Serves 4 • Serving Size: 2 skewers + 1/2 cup rice • Prep Time: 45 minutes

1 pint button mushrooms

1 large zucchini, sliced into 1/2-inch thick rounds

1 large yellow squash, sliced into 1/2-inch thick rounds

2 red bell peppers, sliced into 1-inch chunks

2 lb beef tenderloin, cut into 1-inch cubes

8 bamboo skewers, soaked in warm water

2 Tbsp lite soy sauce

2 Tbsp rice wine vinegar

2 tsp sesame oil

1 clove garlic, minced

4 green onions, chopped

2 cups cooked brown rice

Nutrition Tip:
Kabobs are a great way to get protein and vegetable servings in one easy dish.

1. Prepare indoor or outdoor grill.

Exchanges/Choices
1 1/2 Starch
2 Vegetable
6 Lean Meat
1 Fat

Calories	475
Calories from Fat	135
Total Fat	15 g
Saturated Fat	5 g
Trans Fat	0 g
Cholesterol	115 mg
Sodium	395 mg
Total Carbohydrate	36 g
Dietary Fiber	6 g
Sugars	8 g
Protein	49 g

2. Assemble kabobs by alternating mushrooms, zucchini, squash, peppers, and beef on each skewer (making eight skewers).

3. In a medium bowl, whisk together soy sauce, rice wine vinegar, sesame oil, garlic, and green onions. Pour into a large sealable plastic bag.

4. Place kabobs in plastic bag with marinade. Shake until all kabobs are coated; marinate in the refrigerator for 30 minutes.

5. Grill over medium heat for 10 minutes, turning occasionally.

6. Serve kabobs over brown rice.

BACON CHEESE TURKEY BURGER

Serves 5 • Serving Size: 1 burger • Prep Time: 15 minutes

1 1/4 lb lean ground turkey breast

1/3 cup reduced-fat, shredded cheddar cheese

5 slices turkey bacon, cooked and cut into 1/2-inch pieces

1 tsp grill seasoning

5 whole-wheat hamburger buns

5 tomato slices

5 lettuce leaves

1. Prepare an indoor or outdoor grill.

2. In a medium bowl, combine the turkey, cheese, bacon, and grill seasoning. Divide into five equal portions, shaping into 1/2-inch thick patties.

3. Place patties on grill rack and grill 7 minutes on each side or until done.

4. Serve on buns, with a tomato slice and a lettuce leaf.

Nutrition Tip:
Who says you can never eat a bacon cheeseburger if you have diabetes? With a few low-fat substitutions, this recipe proves that healthy eating does not have to be boring and tasteless.

Exchanges/Choices
1 1/2 Starch
4 Lean Meat

Calories	295
Calories from Fat	65
Total Fat	7 g
Saturated Fat	2.3 g
Trans Fat	0 g
Cholesterol	90 mg
Sodium	485 mg
Total Carbohydrate	23 g
Dietary Fiber	4 g
Sugars	5 g
Protein	35 g

BAKED PENNE
WITH VEGETABLES

Serves 10 • Serving Size: 1/10th recipe • Prep Time: 25 minutes

Cooking spray

13.25-oz box whole-wheat penne pasta, uncooked

1 Tbsp olive oil

1 green pepper, diced

3 cups mushrooms, sliced

3 zucchini, diced

3 garlic cloves, minced

1 1 lb, 10-oz jar pasta sauce

1 14.5-oz can no-salt-added diced tomato

1 1/2 cups part-skim, shredded mozzarella cheese

2 Tbsp grated Parmesan cheese

Cooking Tip:
This pasta would be wonderful served along with baked chicken or pork. It works great for a dinner party because it makes a large amount.

1. Preheat oven to 350°F. Spray a 9 × 13-inch baking dish with cooking spray. Cook pasta according to package directions, omitting salt. Drain.

2. Spray a large sauté pan with cooking spray, add oil, and heat over medium-high heat. Add green pepper, mushrooms, and zucchini, and sauté for 7–10 minutes. Add garlic and sauté 30 seconds.

3. In large bowl, combine cooked pasta, vegetables, pasta sauce, and diced tomatoes. Mix well.

4. Pour pasta mixture into a baking dish. Top with mozzarella and Parmesan cheese. Bake 25 minutes.

Exchanges/Choices
2 1/2 Starch
1 Vegetable
1/2 Fat

Calories	255
Calories from Fat	45
Total Fat	5 g
Saturated Fat	2.2 g
Trans Fat	0 g
Cholesterol	10 mg
Sodium	375 mg
Total Carbohydrate	42 g
Dietary Fiber	7 g
Sugars	8 g
Protein	13 g

BAKED TILAPIA

Serves 4 • Serving Size: 1 fillet • Prep Time: 5 minutes

Cooking spray
1/4 cup light mayonnaise
1/4 cup grated fat-free Parmesan cheese
3 Tbsp fresh dill, chopped
4 tilapia fillets (1 1/4 lb total)
2 cups cooked brown rice

1. Preheat oven to 375°F. Coat a baking dish with cooking spray.

2. In a small bowl, combine the mayonnaise, Parmesan cheese, and dill.

3. Coat each fillet with the mayonnaise mixture. Place fillets in baking dish and bake 18–20 minutes.

4. Serve hot with 1/2 cup rice.

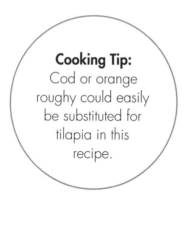

Cooking Tip:
Cod or orange roughy could easily be substituted for tilapia in this recipe.

Exchanges/Choices
2 Starch
4 Lean Meat

Calories 325
  Calories from Fat.....80
Total Fat ....9 g
  Saturated Fat ....2.2 g
  Trans Fat ....0 g
Cholesterol ....100 mg
Sodium ....275 mg
Total Carbohydrate ....27 g
  Dietary Fiber ....2 g
  Sugars ....2 g
Protein.....................33 g

BBQ CHICKEN PIZZA MEAL

Serves 8 • Serving Size: 1 slice • Prep Time: 25 minutes

Pizza

Cooking spray

1/2 lb boneless skinless chicken breast, cooked

1/4 tsp salt (*optional*)

1/4 tsp ground black pepper

1/4 cup sugar-free orange marmalade

1/4 cup barbeque sauce

1/2 tsp hot sauce

1 (12-inch) prepackaged whole-wheat Italian pizza crust

1/2 medium red onion, diced small

3/4 cup reduced-fat, shredded mozzarella cheese

Salad

8 cups salad greens mix

16 tomato slices

1 cup diced cucumber

7 Tbsp fat-free Italian salad dressing

1. Preheat oven to 375°F. Spray a baking sheet with cooking spray.

2. Season chicken with salt (optional) and pepper on both sides.

3. Place chicken on prepared baking sheet and bake for 25 minutes or until juices run clear; chop chicken into half-inch pieces.

4. In a small saucepan, combine sugar-free orange marmalade, barbeque sauce, and hot sauce. Bring to a boil.

Cooking Tip:
The whole-wheat Italian pizza crust is a fairly new product and is found along with the regular Italian pizza crust at most grocery stores.

5. Spoon sauce over pizza crust. Top crust with cooked chicken, diced onion, and mozzarella cheese.

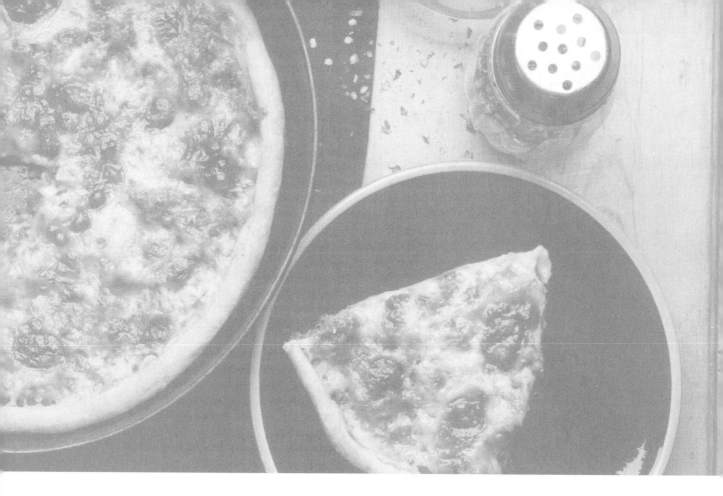

6. Bake on rack for 20–25 minutes or until cheese is melted and bubbly.

7. While the pizza bakes, prepare the eight individual side salads (1 cup greens, 2 tomato slices, 2 Tbsp diced cucumber, and 1 Tbsp dressing).

Exchanges/Choices
1 Starch
1/2 Carbohydrate
1 Vegetable
1 Lean Meat
1/2 Fat

Calories	210
Calories from Fat	40
Total Fat	4.5 g
Saturated Fat	2.1 g
Trans Fat	0 g
Cholesterol	20 mg
Sodium	510 mg
Total Carbohydrate	30 g
Dietary Fiber	4 g
Sugars	9 g
Protein	14 g

BEEF AND ASPARAGUS ROLL UPS

Serves 4 • Serving Size: 3 pieces + 1/2 cup rice • Prep Time: 10 minutes

Cooking spray

1 lb asparagus, trimmed to 3-inch pieces (about 24 pieces)

1 lb beef sirloin steak, pounded thin

2 Tbsp lite soy sauce

1 Tbsp sesame oil

1 Tbsp sesame seeds

2 cups cooked brown rice

Cooking Tip:
Check the meat case in your grocery store for "sandwich" steak. It is sirloin steak that has been pounded thin, saving you a cooking step.

1. Preheat oven to 400°F. Coat a baking sheet with cooking spray.

2. Bring a large saucepan of water to a boil. Add asparagus to boiling water and boil for 1 minute to blanch. Remove asparagus and set aside to cool.

3. Slice pounded steak into 12 equal-sized strips.

4. Take two pieces of asparagus and lay together at one end of a beef strip. Roll up and place seam side down on prepared baking sheet. Repeat for remaining 11 beef strips.

5. In a small bowl, whisk soy sauce and sesame oil. Brush mixture evenly over beef roll ups. Sprinkle sesame seeds evenly over roll ups.

6. Bake in oven for 7 minutes. Turn oven up to broil and place baking sheet under broiler for 3 minutes. Serve roll ups over 1/2 cup cooked brown rice.

Exchanges/Choices	
1 1/2 Starch	
1 Vegetable	
3 Lean Meat	
1 Fat	
Calories	305
Calories from Fat	90
Total Fat	10 g
Saturated Fat	2.4 g
Trans Fat	0.1 g
Cholesterol	40 mg
Sodium	155 mg
Total Carbohydrate	27 g
Dietary Fiber	3 g
Sugars	2 g
Protein	28 g

BEEF AND BARLEY STEW

Serves 5 • Serving Size: 1 cup • Prep Time: 10 minutes

1 Tbsp olive oil

1/2 lb lean sirloin steak, cut into small chunks

1 medium onion, diced

3 medium carrots, diced

2 medium celery stalks, diced

1 medium sweet potato, diced

1 32-oz can reduced-sodium, fat-free beef broth

1 cup instant barley

1/2 tsp salt (*optional*)

1/2 tsp ground black pepper

1/2 tsp onion powder

1 tsp cornstarch

2 Tbsp cold water

1. Add oil to a large soup pot and heat over medium-high heat.

2. Add beef and sauté for 2 minutes. Remove from pot, set aside. Add onions, carrots, celery, and sweet potato to pot and sauté 6–7 minutes or until ingredients begin to caramelize.

3. Add broth, barley, salt (optional), pepper, and onion powder. Reduce heat and simmer for 20 minutes.

4. In a small bowl, whisk together cornstarch and water. Add to stew and bring to a boil. Remove from heat; stir in beef and remaining juices.

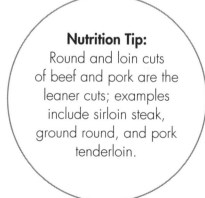

Nutrition Tip:
Round and loin cuts of beef and pork are the leaner cuts; examples include sirloin steak, ground round, and pork tenderloin.

Exchanges/Choices	
2 Starch	
1 Vegetable	
1 Lean Meat	
1/2 Fat	

Calories	250
Calories from Fat	45
Total Fat	5 g
Saturated Fat	1.1 g
Trans Fat	0.1 g
Cholesterol	15 mg
Sodium	400 mg
Total Carbohydrate	37 g
Dietary Fiber	5 g
Sugars	5 g
Protein	15 g

the healthy carb diabetes cookbook

BEEF STIR-FRY

Serves 5 • Serving Size: 1/5th recipe • Prep Time: 15 minutes

2 1/2 cups cooked brown rice

Cooking spray

1 lb boneless eye or round steak, cut into
 1-inch strips

1 cup snow peas, trimmed

1 medium red pepper, cut into strips

2 cups shredded carrots

2 cups sliced mushrooms

1 tsp Chinese five-spice powder

1 cup reduced-sodium, fat-free beef broth

1 1/2 Tbsp lite soy sauce

1 dash cayenne pepper (*optional*)

1 Tbsp cornstarch

Cooking Tip:
If you don't have
Chinese five-spice powder,
you can substitute equal parts
ground cinnamon, ground
cloves, ground fennel seeds,
ground anise, and
ground pepper.

1. Cook rice according to package directions.

Exchanges/Choices
1 1/2 Starch
2 Vegetable
3 Lean Meat

Calories	275
Calories from Fat	35
Total Fat	4 g
Saturated Fat	1.3 g
Trans Fat	0 g
Cholesterol	40 mg
Sodium	330 mg
Total Carbohydrate	33 g
Dietary Fiber	4 g
Sugars	5 g
Protein	26 g

2. Coat a nonstick sauté pan or wok with cooking spray and sauté steak over high heat. Remove steak from pan and set aside, reserving juices.

3. Sauté snow peas, red pepper, carrots, and mushrooms for 4 minutes. Add steak and juices back to pan.

4. In a small bowl, whisk together remaining ingredients. Pour mixture over stir-fry. Bring to a boil and reduce to a simmer for 2–3 minutes. Serve over rice.

BEEF TACO SUPREME

Serves 9 • Serving Size: 1 taco • Prep Time: 10 minutes

1 lb 90% lean ground beef

2/3 cup water

1 tsp cumin

1 Tbsp chili powder

1/4 tsp cayenne powder

1 tsp onion powder

1 cup canned black beans, rinsed and drained

9 whole-wheat tortillas, warmed*

1/2 avocado, diced

1 cup lettuce, shredded

1 large tomato, diced

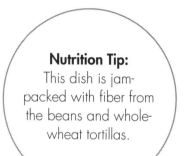

Nutrition Tip:
This dish is jam-packed with fiber from the beans and whole-wheat tortillas.

1. Brown the beef in large nonstick skillet over medium-high heat until thoroughly cooked and no longer pink. Drain fat.

2. Add water, cumin, chili powder, cayenne pepper, and onion powder; simmer for 5 minutes or until all liquid is absorbed.

3. Add beans and heat an additional 3 minutes.

4. Fill each tortilla with 1/4 cup meat and bean mixture, spoonful of avocado, lettuce, and tomato.

*Each tortilla should have 30 g carbohydrate and 4 g dietary fiber per serving.

Exchanges/Choices
2 Starch
2 Lean Meat
1 Fat

Calories 295	
Calories from Fat.....80	
Total Fat ....9 g	
Saturated Fat ....2.1 g	
Trans Fat ....0.3 g	
Cholesterol ....30 mg	
Sodium ....455 mg	
Total Carbohydrate ....35 g	
Dietary Fiber ....7 g	
Sugars ....3 g	
Protein ....16 g	

BREADED PORK MEDALLIONS WITH CRANBERRY ONION CHUTNEY

Serves 8 • Serving Size: 2 medallions • Prep Time: 15 minutes

Cranberry Onion Chutney

2 tsp olive oil

1/2 medium red onion, diced

1 cup fresh cranberries

1/4 cup Splenda

1/2 cup balsamic vinegar

1/2 cup low-sugar apricot preserves

Breaded Pork Medallions

1 lb pork tenderloin, cut into 16 medallions

3 egg whites

1 tsp hot sauce

3/4 cup cornmeal

1/2 tsp garlic salt

1/2 tsp ground black pepper

2 tsp olive oil

Cooking spray

Cooking Tip:
If you can't find fresh, whole cranberries, check the frozen section. Be sure to buy fresh-frozen berries and not ones packed in syrup or added sugar.

1. Heat a medium saucepan over medium high heat. Add olive oil and red onion, and sauté 6–7 minutes or until ingredients begin to caramelize. Add cranberries, Splenda, vinegar, and preserves. Bring to a boil. Reduce to a simmer and cook for 15 minutes or until chutney has a thick jam-like consistency.

2. Pound pork medallions until about 1/4 inch thick.

3. In a small bowl, whisk together egg whites and hot sauce. In a separate bowl, stir together the cornmeal, garlic salt, and black pepper.

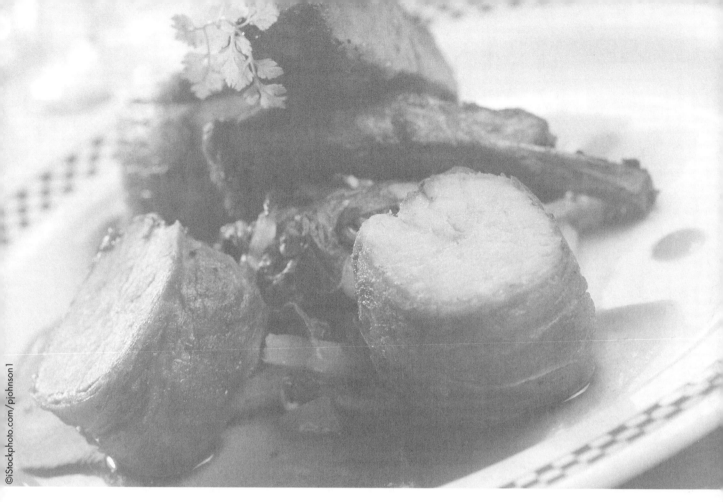

4. Dip each medallion in egg mixture, then in cornmeal to coat.

5. Heat a large sauté pan over medium-high heat. Add olive oil and a generous amount of cooking spray to the pan. Once the oil is hot, sauté the medallions in batches, cooking for about 2 minutes on each side.

6. Serve chutney over the medallions.

Exchanges/Choices
1 1/2 Carbohydrate
2 Lean Meat

Calories 180
  Calories from Fat..... 35
Total Fat .... 4 g
  Saturated Fat .... 0.8 g
  Trans Fat .... 0 g
Cholesterol .... 30 mg
Sodium .... 125 mg
Total Carbohydrate .... 22 g
  Dietary Fiber .... 2 g
  Sugars .... 9 g
Protein .... 13 g

BROWN RICE AND MUSHROOM STUFFED CHICKEN BREAST

Serves 4 • Serving Size: 1 chicken breast • Prep Time: 15 minutes

1 tsp olive oil

1 cup mushrooms, diced

3 Tbsp slivered almonds

1 cup water

1/2 cup instant brown rice

4 4-oz boneless, skinless chicken breasts

1/4 tsp salt (*optional*)

1/2 tsp ground black pepper

1 tsp dried thyme

Cooking spray

1. Preheat oven to 350°F.

2. In a medium saucepan, heat oil over medium-high heat. Add mushrooms; sauté 4–5 minutes. Add almonds and sauté 2 more minutes.

3. Add water and brown rice to saucepan and bring to a boil. Reduce heat; cover and simmer for 10 minutes (or according to rice package directions).

Cooking Tip:
If you have any rice left over from this recipe, serve chicken breast on a small bed of rice.

4. Place one chicken breast on a cutting board and cover with plastic wrap. Pound meat with a meat tenderizer or rolling pin until it is about 1/4 inch thick. Repeat this process for the other three breasts. Set aside.

5. Spread 1/4 cup rice mixture on one side of the pounded chicken breast. Roll breast and secure the seam with a toothpick. Repeat procedure for remaining three chicken breasts.

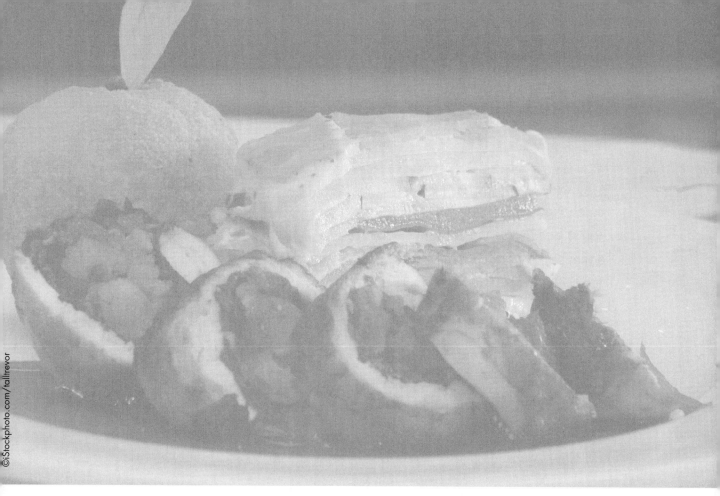

6. Sprinkle all sides of rolled chicken breasts with equal amounts of salt (optional), pepper, and thyme. Coat a glass or metal baking dish with cooking spray and place chicken in dish seam side down. Bake for 30 minutes or until chicken is done.

7. To serve, remove toothpicks and slice each piece into five rounds.

Exchanges/Choices
1 1/2 Starch
3 Lean Meat
1/2 Fat

Calories	260
Calories from Fat	70
Total Fat	8 g
Saturated Fat	1.2 g
Trans Fat	0 g
Cholesterol	65 mg
Sodium	70 mg
Total Carbohydrate	20 g
Dietary Fiber	2 g
Sugars	1 g
Protein	28 g

BUTTERNUT SQUASH PASTA

Serves 9 • Serving Size: 1 cup • Prep Time: 15 minutes

16 oz whole-wheat rotini pasta, uncooked

1 large butternut squash (about 2 lb)

Cooking spray

1 tsp olive oil

8 oz fat-free ricotta cheese

3/4 cup nonfat milk

4 oz light cream cheese, cubed

1/4 cup grated Parmesan cheese

1/4 tsp cayenne pepper

1/4 tsp salt (*optional*)

1/4 tsp ground black pepper

1/8 tsp ground nutmeg

1. Cook pasta according to package directions, omitting salt. Drain.

2. Preheat oven to 400°F.

3. Spray both sides of squash with cooking spray and place face down in a glass baking dish. Bake for 45–50 minutes, until soft.

4. Remove squash from oven. Scoop squash meat into a large bowl. Set aside.

5. In a large saucepan, heat olive oil, ricotta cheese, milk, and cream cheese over low heat until cheese is melted. Add cooked squash and remaining ingredients; whisk until smooth and cook until thoroughly heated.

6. Add cooked pasta to pan and toss gently to coat.

Exchanges/Choices
3 Starch
1 Fat

Calories 275
    Calories from Fat.....45
Total Fat ....5 g
    Saturated Fat.............2.4 g
    Trans Fat ....0 g
Cholesterol ....20 mg
Sodium ....110 mg
Total Carbohydrate ....48 g
    Dietary Fiber ....5 g
    Sugars ....5 g
Protein....................14 g

Cooking Tip:
This recipe is perfect for a cool autumn day. If you'd like some protein with it, pork tenderloin works well.

CAJUN SHRIMP SKEWERS

Serves 9 • Serving Size: 1 skewer • Prep Time: 10 minutes

1 1/2 Tbsp olive oil
1 tsp Cajun seasoning
1 lb raw medium shrimp, peeled and deveined
9 bamboo skewers, soaked in warm water

1. Prepare an indoor or outdoor grill.

2. In a medium bowl, whisk together olive oil and Cajun seasoning. Add shrimp to bowl and toss to coat evenly.

3. Divide shrimp evenly among nine skewers.

4. Grill skewers 2–3 minutes on each side or until shrimp are pink and slightly firm to the touch.

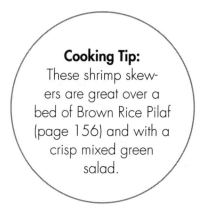

Cooking Tip:
These shrimp skewers are great over a bed of Brown Rice Pilaf (page 156) and with a crisp mixed green salad.

Exchanges/Choices
1 Lean Meat

Calories	50
Calories from Fat	20
Total Fat	2.5 g
Saturated Fat	0.4 g
Trans Fat	0 g
Cholesterol	60 mg
Sodium	95 mg
Total Carbohydrate	0 g
Dietary Fiber	0 g
Sugars	0 g
Protein	6 g

CARIBBEAN CHICKEN WITH SWEET POTATOES

Serves 4 • Serving Size: 1 breast + 1 cup potato mix • Prep Time: 15 minutes

3 Tbsp Splenda Brown Sugar Blend

1/2 tsp cayenne pepper (1/4 tsp if you prefer less spicy)

1/2 tsp ground nutmeg

1/2 tsp ground cinnamon

1/2 tsp ground black pepper

1 Tbsp dried thyme

2 tsp water

4 4-oz boneless, skinless chicken breasts

1 Tbsp canola oil

1 medium onion, diced

2 cloves garlic, minced

1 14.5-oz can no-salt-added diced tomatoes

2 large sweet potatoes (about 1 lb), halved lengthwise and sliced into 1/2-inch half moons

1 1/2 cups reduced-sodium, fat-free chicken broth

1. In a small bowl, combine the Splenda Brown Sugar Blend, cayenne, nutmeg, cinnamon, black pepper, thyme, and water. Rub mixture evenly over breasts.

2. Heat oil in a large sauté pan over medium-low heat. Add chicken and cook 8 minutes per side. Remove chicken from pan.

3. Turn heat up to medium, add onion and cook additional 2 minutes, and add garlic and cook 1 additional minute.

4. Add tomatoes, sweet potatoes, and chicken broth to pan and bring the liquid to a boil. Reduce heat and simmer uncovered, until the sweet potatoes are tender (about 40 minutes). Add chicken back to pan and cook 5 minutes until heated through.

Exchanges/Choices
1 1/2 Starch
1/2 Carbohydrate
2 Vegetable
3 Lean Meat

Calories	350
Calories from Fat	65
Total Fat	7 g
Saturated Fat	1.2 g
Trans Fat	0 g
Cholesterol	65 mg
Sodium	300 mg
Total Carbohydrate	44 g
Dietary Fiber	5 g
Sugars	20 g
Protein	28 g

Nutrition Tip:
One-pot meals can provide a healthy meal with a variety of food groups. This recipe gives you protein and vegetables.

CARNE ASADA TACOS

Serves 8 • Serving Size: 2 tacos • Prep Time: 55 minutes

1 lime, juiced

3 cloves garlic, minced

2 green onions, chopped

1 lb flank steak

1 Tbsp canola oil

16 small whole-wheat tortillas (about 6 inches in diameter each)

1. Preheat oven to 375°F.

2. In a small bowl, whisk together lime juice, garlic, and green onions. Pour into a large sealable bag. Add steak, seal, and marinate in refrigerator for 45 minutes.

3. Add oil to a medium oven-safe skillet and heat over high heat. Remove steak from marinade and sear on one side for 2 minutes. Flip steak, pour marinade over it, and bake in oven for 10–15 minutes.

4. Remove steak from oven and let rest for 5 minutes. Slice meat thinly against the grain. Divide meat among whole-wheat tortillas.

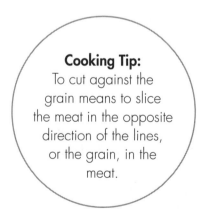

Cooking Tip:
To cut against the grain means to slice the meat in the opposite direction of the lines, or the grain, in the meat.

Exchanges/Choices
2 Starch
2 Lean Meat
1/2 Fat

Calories	260
Calories from Fat	70
Total Fat	8 g
Saturated Fat	1.6 g
Trans Fat	0 g
Cholesterol	20 mg
Sodium	415 mg
Total Carbohydrate	29 g
Dietary Fiber	4 g
Sugars	2 g
Protein	15 g

CHICKEN ALMOND STIR-FRY

Serves 6 • Serving Size: 1 cup stir-fry + 1/3 cup rice • Prep Time: 15 minutes

Cooking spray

1 Tbsp canola oil

3 cups broccoli florets

1 cup sugar snap peas

2 cups baby carrots

2 4-oz boneless, skinless chicken breasts, cut into 1-inch strips

2 tsp lite soy sauce

1/2 tsp garlic powder

1/4 tsp ground black pepper

2 Tbsp sliced almonds

2 cups cooked brown rice

1. Add cooking spray and canola oil to a large nonstick skillet or wok over medium-high heat. Add broccoli, sugar snap peas, and carrots, and stir-fry for 4 minutes.

2. Add chicken, soy sauce, garlic powder, and pepper to skillet and stir-fry for 6 more minutes or until chicken is cooked through. Add almonds and sauté 1 minute.

3. Serve stir-fry over rice.

Exchanges/Choices
1 Starch
1 Vegetable
1 Lean Meat
1 Fat

Calories	190
Calories from Fat	55
Total Fat	6 g
Saturated Fat	0.7 g
Trans Fat	0 g
Cholesterol	20 mg
Sodium	125 mg
Total Carbohydrate	23 g
Dietary Fiber	4 g
Sugars	4 g
Protein	12 g

Cooking Tip:
For a timesaver, you can use a bag of mixed pre-cut vegetables, available in the produce section.

CHICKEN AND CORN STEW

Serves 8 • Serving Size: 1 cup • Prep Time: 15 minutes

1 Tbsp olive oil

1 lb boneless, skinless chicken breast, cut into small chunks

1 cup diced carrots

1 cup diced celery

1 cup diced onion

1 tsp garlic powder

1 tsp dried thyme

1 lb frozen corn niblets

1 15.8-oz can navy beans, rinsed and drained

32 oz reduced-sodium, fat-free chicken broth

3/4 cup quick barley

2 bay leaves

1/2 tsp salt (*optional*)

1/2 tsp ground black pepper

1. Add olive oil to a large soup pot over medium-high heat. Add chicken and sauté for 3–4 minutes or until it begins to cook through.

2. Add carrots, celery, and onion. Saute for 5 minutes or until onions turn clear and chicken is cooked.

3. Add remaining ingredients. Bring to a boil, then reduce to a simmer for 20 minutes.

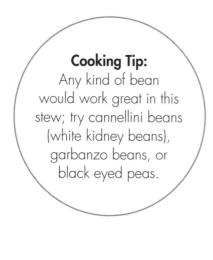

Cooking Tip:
Any kind of bean would work great in this stew; try cannellini beans (white kidney beans), garbanzo beans, or black eyed peas.

Exchanges/Choices
2 Starch
1 Vegetable
2 Lean Meat

Calories 250
   Calories from Fat.....35
Total Fat....................4 g
   Saturated Fat............0.7 g
   Trans Fat ....0 g
Cholesterol ....35 mg
Sodium ....375 mg
Total Carbohydrate....36 g
   Dietary Fiber ....6 g
   Sugars ....4 g
Protein....................20 g

CHICKEN AND NOODLE CASSEROLE

Serves 7 • Serving Size: 1 cup • Prep Time: 20 minutes

Cooking spray

2 Tbsp canola oil

1 medium onion, peeled and diced

3 cups diced, cooked chicken

2 cups frozen mixed vegetables

1 8-oz can water chestnuts, drained and chopped

1 10 3/4-oz can low-fat condensed cream of chicken soup

1/4 cup light mayonnaise

1/4 cup fat-free sour cream

1 cup cooked whole-wheat macaroni noodles

1/8 tsp ground black pepper

1/4 cup reduced-fat, shredded cheddar cheese

Cooking Tip:
Half a cup of uncooked macaroni noodles will result in 1 cup cooked noodles.

Exchanges/Choices
1 Starch
2 Vegetable
2 Lean Meat
1 1/2 Fat

Calories 285
   Calories from Fat...100
Total Fat ....11 g
   Saturated Fat ....2.3 g
   Trans Fat ....0 g
Cholesterol ....60 mg
Sodium ....380 mg
Total Carbohydrate ....22 g
   Dietary Fiber ....3 g
   Sugars ....5 g
Protein ....24 g

1. Preheat oven to 350°F. Coat a 3-quart casserole dish with cooking spray.

2. Heat oil in a small skillet over medium heat. Add onion and sauté until translucent, about 5 minutes. Remove from heat and transfer to a large bowl.

3. Add all remaining ingredients, except cheese, to bowl. Mix together until thoroughly combined.

4. Pour mixture into casserole dish, sprinkle with cheese. Bake for 20–25 minutes or until bubbly. Let stand for a few minutes before serving.

CHICKEN AND TOAST

Serves 4 • Serving Size: 1 cup + 1 piece of toast • Prep Time: 15 minutes

1 Tbsp olive oil

Cooking spray

1 medium onion, diced

1 cup diced carrot

5 cups fresh spinach

1 lb boneless, skinless chicken breast, diced

1 tsp garlic powder

1/2 tsp ground black pepper

1 10 3/4-oz can low-fat condensed cream of celery soup

1 cup reduced-sodium, fat-free chicken broth

4 pieces whole-wheat bread, toasted

Nutrition Tip:
This one-pot meal has real comfort food taste, without the high-fat and high-carb ingredients.

1. Add oil and a generous amount of cooking spray to a large, deep skillet over medium-high heat. Add onion, carrot, and spinach, and sauté for 4–5 minutes or until carrots begin to soften.

2. Add chicken and continue to sauté 3–4 more minutes.

3. Add garlic powder, ground black pepper, soup, and broth. Bring to a boil. Reduce heat to a simmer and cook for 5 minutes.

4. Serve 1 cup of chicken mixture over 1 slice whole-wheat toast.

This recipe is high in sodium.

Exchanges/Choices	
1 Starch	
2 Vegetable	
3 Lean Meat	
1 Fat	

Calories	320
Calories from Fat	80
Total Fat	9 g
Saturated Fat	2.7 g
Trans Fat	0 g
Cholesterol	70 mg
Sodium	915 mg
Total Carbohydrate	27 g
Dietary Fiber	4 g
Sugars	6 g
Protein	31 g

CHICKEN PICATTA PASTA

Serves 7 • Serving Size: 1 cup • Prep Time: 20 minutes

2 cups whole-wheat penne pasta, uncooked

3 4-oz boneless, skinless chicken breast
halves, cut into 1-inch strips

1/2 tsp ground black pepper

2 Tbsp olive oil

1 cup reduced-sodium, fat-free chicken broth

1 lemon, juiced

1 Tbsp cornstarch

1 clove garlic, minced

1 Tbsp bottled capers, rinsed and drained

1/4 cup Italian (flat leaf) parsley, chopped

Cooking Tip:
Italian parsley is
also called flat leaf
parsley. It looks a lot like
cilantro, so be sure you
don't mix up the two!

1. Cook pasta according to package directions, omitting salt. Drain.

2. Season chicken with black pepper.

3. Heat olive oil in a large nonstick skillet over medium-high heat. Add chicken and cook for about 5 minutes or until done. Remove chicken from pan.

4. Add the chicken broth, lemon juice, cornstarch, and garlic to pan; increase heat to high and bring to a boil. Reduce heat and simmer for 3 minutes. Return the chicken to skillet and add capers. Simmer for about 2 minutes or until sauce has thickened.

5. Pour chicken and sauce over cooked pasta and toss. Top with chopped parsley and serve.

Exchanges/Choices
1 Starch
2 Lean Meat

Calories 180
   Calories from Fat..... 45
Total Fat .... 5 g
   Saturated Fat .... 0.9 g
   Trans Fat .... 0 g
Cholesterol .... 30 mg
Sodium .... 135 mg
Total Carbohydrate .... 19 g
   Dietary Fiber .... 3 g
   Sugars .... 1 g
Protein .... 14 g

CHIPOTLE PORK ENCHILADAS

Serves 5 • Serving Size: 2 enchiladas • Prep Time: 15 minutes

1 Tbsp olive oil

3/4 lb lean pork, diced

1 chipotle pepper in adobo sauce
from can, chopped

1 tsp chili powder

1 tsp cumin

1 14.5-oz can fat-free refried beans

Cooking spray

10 (6-inch) corn tortillas

1/2 cup reduced-fat, shredded
cheddar cheese

Sauce

2 8-oz cans no-salt-added tomato
sauce

1 Tbsp adobo sauce (from canned
chipotle pepper)

1 tsp cumin

Cooking Tip:
Chipotle peppers in
adobo sauce are spicy.
If you like your food a
less spicy, use half the
amount called for in
the recipe.

1. Preheat oven to 350°F.

2. Add olive oil to a medium sauté pan over medium-high heat.

3. Add pork and sauté 2–3 minutes. Add chipotle pepper, chili powder, cumin, and refried beans. Sauté 2 more minutes.

4. In a medium bowl, combine tomato sauce, adobo sauce, and cumin.

5. Spray a 9 × 13-inch baking dish with cooking spray. Fill each tortilla with a portion of the pork mixture (divided evenly among the 10 tortillas). Roll tortillas and place seam side down in the pan. Pour sauce over tortillas and distribute evenly. Top with cheese. Bake for 20 minutes.

Exchanges/Choices
2 Starch
1 Vegetable
2 Lean Meat
1 1/2 Fat

Calories 355
  Calories from Fat...100
Total Fat ....11 g
  Saturated Fat ....3.5 g
  Trans Fat ....0 g
Cholesterol ....45 mg
Sodium ....530 mg
Total Carbohydrate ....41 g
  Dietary Fiber ....8 g
  Sugars ....7 g
Protein ....23 g

CREAMY TILAPIA BAKE

Serves 4 • Serving Size: 1 fillet • Prep Time: 10 minutes

Cooking spray

1 10.75-oz can cream of shrimp soup

1/2 cup nonfat milk

2 cups cooked brown rice

4 tilapia fillets (about 1/4 lb each)

2 tsp paprika

1/4 tsp ground black pepper

1. Preheat oven to 350°F.

2. Spray a 9 × 13-inch baking dish with cooking spray.

3. In a small bowl, whisk together soup and nonfat milk.

4. Spread cooked rice evenly over the bottom of the baking pan. Lay the tilapia fillets across the rice. Do not overlap.

5. Pour soup and milk mixture over the fish and sprinkle with paprika and pepper.

6. Bake for 15 minutes or until bubbly.

Exchanges/Choices
1 1/2 Starch
1/2 Carbohydrate
3 Lean Meat

Calories 290
   Calories from Fat.....65
Total Fat ....7 g
   Saturated Fat.............1.8 g
   Trans Fat ....0 g
Cholesterol ....85 mg
Sodium ....600 mg
Total Carbohydrate ....30 g
   Dietary Fiber ....3 g
   Sugars ....2 g
Protein ....27 g

Cooking Tip:
If you can't find cream of shrimp soup, try cream of celery.

CUBAN PORK TENDERLOIN

Serves 8 • Serving Size: 1/8th recipe • Prep Time: 35 minutes

4 limes, juiced

1 small orange, juiced

3 garlic cloves, minced

2 lb pork tenderloin, trimmed of all fat
   (2 1-lb pork tenderloins can be used)

1 tsp dried oregano

1/2 tsp salt (*optional*)

1/4 tsp ground black pepper

1/2 tsp cumin

Cooking spray

Cooking Tip:
This pork tastes great served with a side of sweet potatoes—try it with the Sweet Potatoes with Brown Sugar Glaze on page 191.

1. In a large bowl, add lime juice, orange juice, and garlic. Marinate pork in this mixture for 30 minutes in refrigerator.

2. Preheat oven to 375°F.

3. Remove pork from marinade and rub with oregano, salt (optional), pepper, and cumin.

4. Coat a large oven-safe sauté pan with cooking spray. Heat over high heat. Add pork tenderloin and sear on each side for 3 minutes.

5. Pour remaining marinade over pork.

6. Place pan in oven and bake for 40–50 minutes or until done.

7. Remove pork from pan and set on cutting board to rest for 5 minutes before slicing.

Exchanges/Choices
3 Lean Meat

Calories	125
Calories from Fat	25
Total Fat	3 g
Saturated Fat	1 g
Trans Fat	0 g
Cholesterol	60 mg
Sodium	45 mg
Total Carbohydrate	2 g
Dietary Fiber	0 g
Sugars	1 g
Protein	22 g

CURRY BEEF WITH BROWN RICE

Serves 4 • Serving Size: 1/2 cup rice + 1/2 heaping cup stir-fry • Prep Time: 10 minutes

1 Tbsp olive oil

1 lb sirloin beef, sliced and trimmed of all fat

1 cup shredded carrots

1/3 cup green onions, chopped

2 Tbsp raisins

2 cups cooked brown rice

Sauce

1/3 cup plain nonfat yogurt

1/4 cup fat-free half-and-half

2 tsp curry powder

1/4 tsp salt (*optional*)

1/2 tsp ground black pepper

1. Heat oil in a large skillet over high heat. Add beef and sear 2 minutes. Remove beef from skillet and set aside.

2. Add carrots, green onions, and raisins; sauté 2 minutes.

3. In a small bowl, combine sauce ingredients. Add beef and sauce to skillet and simmer for 3–4 minutes. Serve over brown rice.

Exchanges/Choices
1 1/2 Starch
1/2 Carbohydrate
3 Lean Meat
1/2 Fat

Calories 325
  Calories from Fat.....80
Total Fat ....9 g
  Saturated Fat ....2.4 g
  Trans Fat ....0.1 g
Cholesterol ....45 mg
Sodium ....105 mg
Total Carbohydrate ....33 g
  Dietary Fiber ....3 g
  Sugars ....7 g
Protein.....................27 g

Cooking Tip:
Curry powder isn't spicy. If you want, add 1/4 tsp cayenne pepper to this recipe to give it some kick.

FISH NUGGETS

Serves 8 • Serving Size: 5 nuggets • Prep Time: 10 minutes

Cooking spray

3 cups bran flakes, crushed

3 egg whites, beaten

1 tsp hot sauce

2 lb cod fillets, cut into 1-inch squares

1 Tbsp Cajun seasonings

1. Preheat oven to 400°F. Coat a baking sheet with cooking spray.

2. Place bran flakes in a shallow dish.

3. In a bowl, whisk together egg whites and hot sauce.

4. Dip cod fillet squares first in the egg whites and then into the bran flakes.

5. Place the fillet squares on the baking sheet, spray them with cooking spray, and sprinkle with Cajun seasonings.

6. Bake for 15–20 minutes.

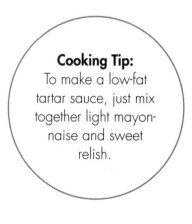

Cooking Tip:
To make a low-fat tartar sauce, just mix together light mayonnaise and sweet relish.

Exchanges/Choices
1 Starch
2 Lean Meat

Calories 160
  Calories from Fat 10
Total Fat .... 1 g
  Saturated Fat .... 0.1 g
  Trans Fat .... 0 g
Cholesterol .... 50 mg
Sodium .... 355 mg
Total Carbohydrate .... 15 g
  Dietary Fiber .... 3 g
  Sugars .... 2 g
Protein .... 24 g

FRENCH ONION SOUP

Serves 8 • Serving Size: 1 cup • Prep Time: 15 minutes

1 Tbsp canola oil

Cooking spray

2 medium onions, thinly sliced

32 oz reduced-sodium, fat-free beef broth

32 oz reduced-sodium, fat-free chicken broth

1/2 tsp dried thyme

1/2 tsp ground black pepper

4 slices whole-wheat bread, crust removed

4 1-oz slices reduced-fat Swiss cheese

Cooking Tip:
To caramelize means to cook the ingredient until it is dark brown but not burned. Stirring frequently while cooking will help evenly caramelize the onions.

1. Preheat oven to 350°F.

2. Heat oil and a generous amount of cooking spray in a soup pot over medium-high heat.

3. Add onions to pot and sauté until completely caramelized, about 20 minutes. Do not burn.

4. Add broths, thyme, and pepper; bring to a boil, then reduce to a simmer for 10 minutes.

5. Coat a baking sheet with cooking spray. Lay bread slices on sheet and top with cheese. If needed, trim the cheese so it is the same size as the slice of bread. Bake for 15 minutes or until cheese is melted and beginning to brown. Remove from oven and cut into 1-inch chunks to make croutons.

6. Pour soup into eight cups and float cheese-and-toast croutons on top of each cup.

Exchanges/Choices
1/2 Carbohydrate
1 Lean Meat
1/2 Fat

Calories	105
Calories from Fat	35
Total Fat	4 g
Saturated Fat	1.2 g
Trans Fat	0 g
Cholesterol	5 mg
Sodium	560 mg
Total Carbohydrate	9 g
Dietary Fiber	1 g
Sugars	2 g
Protein	8 g

GREEK BURGERS

Serves 5 • Serving Size: 1 burger • Prep Time: 10 minutes

1 lb lean ground turkey breast

1/4 cup reduced-fat feta cheese, crumbled

1/2 tsp dried oregano

1/4 tsp ground black pepper

5 tomato slices

5 whole-wheat pita bread pockets

Yogurt Sauce

5 Tbsp nonfat plain yogurt

1 garlic clove, minced

1/2 tsp dried dill

1/2 cucumber, peeled, seeded and grated

1. Prepare an indoor or outdoor grill.

2. In a large bowl, combine ground turkey, feta cheese, oregano, and black pepper. Mix well. Divide into five equal portions and form into 1/2-inch thick patties.

3. Place patties on grill rack and grill for 7 minutes on each side until done (or coat a large nonstick skillet with cooking spray and cook patties over medium heat for 3–4 minutes per side until juices run clear).

4. In a small bowl, combine sauce ingredients.

5. Place one hamburger patty in a pita pocket and top with approximately 1 Tbsp yogurt sauce and one tomato slice. Repeat process for remaining four burgers.

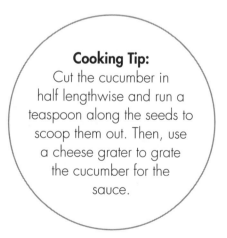

Cooking Tip:
Cut the cucumber in half lengthwise and run a teaspoon along the seeds to scoop them out. Then, use a cheese grater to grate the cucumber for the sauce.

Exchanges/Choices
2 1/2 Starch
2 Lean Meat

Calories	295
Calories from Fat	25
Total Fat	3 g
Saturated Fat	1.1 g
Trans Fat	0 g
Cholesterol	60 mg
Sodium	485 mg
Total Carbohydrate	38 g
Dietary Fiber	5 g
Sugars	2 g
Protein	30 g

INDIAN LAMB-STUFFED TOMATOES

Serves 6 • Serving Size: 1 tomato • Prep Time: 5 minutes

6 large, firm tomatoes (each 3–3 1/2 inches in diameter)

2 Tbsp olive oil

1 large onion, chopped

1 lb lean ground lamb

1/2 cup reduced-sodium, fat-free beef broth

1 Tbsp curry powder

4 Tbsp chopped fresh parsley, divided

1/4 tsp ground cinnamon

3/4 cup cooked brown rice

3 Tbsp freshly grated Parmesan cheese

Cooking Tip:
If you can't find ground lamb in the meat case, ask the butcher to prepare some for you.

1. Preheat oven to 350°F. Cut off top third of tomatoes; chop tops and reserve. Scoop out seeds, juice, and pulp from tomatoes and discard.

2. Add olive oil to a large skillet over medium-high heat. Add onion and sauté until tender and golden, about 8 minutes. Add lamb and sauté until browned, about 7 minutes. Add chopped tomato tops, broth, curry powder, 2 Tbsp parsley, and cinnamon. Bring to a boil. Reduce heat and simmer until mixture thickens, stirring frequently, about 10 minutes. Stir in cooked rice.

3. Place tomatoes in a 13 × 9 × 2-inch glass baking dish. Spoon lamb mixture into the tomatoes. Sprinkle each tomato with Parmesan cheese and remaining parsley.

4. Bake about 25 minutes or until cheese begins to turn golden brown.

Exchanges/Choices
1/2 Starch
2 Vegetable
2 Medium-Fat Meat

Calories	235
Calories from Fat	110
Total Fat	12 g
Saturated Fat	3.4 g
Trans Fat	0 g
Cholesterol	50 mg
Sodium	195 mg
Total Carbohydrate	16 g
Dietary Fiber	3 g
Sugars	6 g
Protein	17 g

ITALIAN MEATLOAF

Serves 6 • Serving Size: 2-inch thick slice • Prep Time: 10 minutes

Cooking spray

1 1/4 lb lean ground turkey breast

1 garlic clove, minced

1 Tbsp dried oregano

1/4 cup fresh Italian parsley, finely chopped

1 tsp dried minced onion

1/4 cup grated Parmesan cheese

1 cup spaghetti sauce, divided

1 egg, slightly beaten

1/2 cup oatmeal

1. Preheat oven to 350°F.

2. Generously coat an 8 1/2-inch loaf pan with cooking spray. In a medium bowl, combine all ingredients; reserving 1/2 cup spaghetti sauce. Mix well.

3. Spread mixture evenly into loaf pan. Top with remaining 1/2 cup spaghetti sauce.

4. Bake for 60 minutes or until no longer pink.

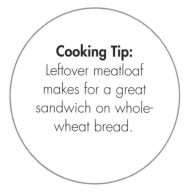

Cooking Tip:
Leftover meatloaf makes for a great sandwich on whole-wheat bread.

Exchanges/Choices
1/2 Starch
3 Lean Meat

Calories 185
   Calories from Fat 25
Total Fat .... 3 g
   Saturated Fat .... 1.2 g
   Trans Fat .... 0 g
Cholesterol .... 95 mg
Sodium .... 225 mg
Total Carbohydrate .... 10 g
   Dietary Fiber .... 2 g
   Sugars .... 3 g
Protein .... 28 g

ITALIAN WEDDING SOUP

Serves 13 • Serving Size: 1 cup • Prep Time: 20 minutes

Meatballs

1 lb lean ground turkey

1 small onion, grated

2 cloves garlic, minced

1 egg

1/4 cup grated Parmesan cheese

2 Tbsp flat leaf parsley, chopped

1/2 tsp ground black pepper

Soup

12 cups reduced-sodium, fat-free chicken broth

4 cups curly endive, stemmed and chopped

1 egg

1 egg white

1/2 tsp salt (*optional*)

1. In a medium bowl, combine meatball ingredients and mix well. Using a tablespoon, form meat into small meatballs.

2. In a large soup pot over high heat, bring chicken broth to a boil; reduce heat to a simmer. Drop meatballs and endive into simmering broth; cook until meatballs are done, about 8–10 minutes.

3. In a small bowl, whisk egg and egg white. Drizzle egg into hot broth, stirring constantly. Season with salt (optional).

Exchanges/Choices
2 Lean Meat

Calories 95
  Calories from Fat 40
Total Fat .... 4.5 g
  Saturated Fat .... 1.6 g
  Trans Fat .... 0 g
Cholesterol .... 65 mg
Sodium .... 535 mg
Total Carbohydrate ...... 3 g
  Dietary Fiber .... 1 g
  Sugars .... 1 g
Protein .... 11 g

Cooking Tip:
For a heartier soup, try adding some barley or whole-wheat elbow macaroni noodles.

JAMBALAYA

Serves 8 • Serving Size: 1/8th recipe • Prep Time: 20 minutes

2 1/2 cups water

1 14-oz can no-salt-added diced tomatoes

1 8-oz can no-salt-added tomato sauce

14 oz lean smoked turkey sausage, cut into chunks

2 4-oz boneless, skinless chicken breasts, cut into chunks

1 cup instant brown rice

3 Tbsp dried minced onion

1/2 tsp dried thyme leaves

1/2 tsp garlic powder

1/2 tsp ground black pepper

1/4 tsp cayenne pepper (optional)

1/4 tsp salt (optional)

1. In a large soup pot, heat the water, tomatoes, tomato sauce, smoked sausage, and chicken breast over medium-high heat. Bring mixture to a boil. Cover, reduce heat, and let simmer for 20 minutes.

2. Add remaining ingredients, simmer for an additional 10 minutes.

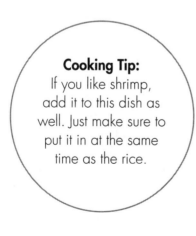

Cooking Tip:
If you like shrimp, add it to this dish as well. Just make sure to put it in at the same time as the rice.

Exchanges/Choices
1 Starch
1 Vegetable
1 Lean Meat

Calories	150
Calories from Fat	20
Total Fat	2 g
Saturated Fat	0.4 g
Trans Fat	0 g
Cholesterol	20 mg
Sodium	180 mg
Total Carbohydrate	25 g
Dietary Fiber	2 g
Sugars	4 g
Protein	9 g

LAMB CHOPS

Serves 4 • Serving Size: 1 chop • Prep Time: 10 minutes

1 tsp curry powder

1 tsp dried oregano

1/4 tsp ground black pepper

4 6-oz lamb loin chops, bone in

1 Tbsp olive oil

1. Preheat oven to 375°F.

2. In a small bowl, combine curry powder, oregano, and ground black pepper. Rub each lamb chop with spice mixture.

3. Add olive oil to a large oven-safe skillet and heat over high heat. Sear each chop on one side for 3–4 minutes or until brown. Turn chops over and place skillet in oven.

4. Cook for an additional 5–6 minutes or until slightly pink in the center.

Exchanges/Choices
3 Lean Meat
1 Fat

Calories	190
Calories from Fat	100
Total Fat	11 g
Saturated Fat	3 g
Trans Fat	0 g
Cholesterol	70 mg
Sodium	60 mg
Total Carbohydrate	1 g
Dietary Fiber	0 g
Sugars	0 g
Protein	22 g

Nutrition Tip:
Sick of chicken? Try the lean cuts of lamb, including loin chops, leg of lamb, and lamb shoulder.

MEDITERRANEAN LENTIL SOUP

Serves 11 • Serving Size: 1 cup • Prep Time: 15 minutes

1 Tbsp olive oil

1 cup celery, diced small

1 medium onion, diced small

2 cloves garlic, minced

10 oz fresh spinach

1 cup dry lentils

Zest of one lemon

Juice of one lemon

1 28-oz can no-salt-added diced tomatoes

80 oz reduced-sodium, fat-free chicken broth

2 cups whole-wheat penne pasta, uncooked

1. In a large stock pot over medium-high heat, add olive oil and sauté celery, onion, garlic, and spinach until onions turn clear. About 5 minutes.

2. Add remaining ingredients, except pasta.

3. Bring to a boil, reduce to simmer, and cook for 40 minutes.

4. Add pasta and cook an additional 10 minutes.

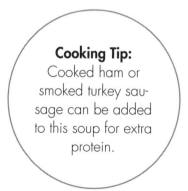

Cooking Tip:
Cooked ham or smoked turkey sausage can be added to this soup for extra protein.

Exchanges/Choices
1 1/2 Starch
1 Vegetable
1/2 Fat

Calories	165
Calories from Fat	20
Total Fat	2 g
Saturated Fat	0.3 g
Trans Fat	0 g
Cholesterol	0 mg
Sodium	560 mg
Total Carbohydrate	28 g
Dietary Fiber	8 g
Sugars	5 g
Protein	10 g

MEDITERRANEAN PIZZA

Serves 8 • Serving Size: 1 slice • Prep Time: 10 minutes

1 (12-inch) prepackaged whole-wheat Italian pizza crust

Olive oil spray

2 garlic cloves, minced

4 plum (roma) tomatoes, cut into chunks

3 Tbsp fresh basil, chopped

1 Tbsp capers

1/3 cup reduced-fat feta cheese, crumbled

1. Preheat oven to 375°F.

2. Spray pizza crust with olive oil spray. Sprinkle minced garlic on top. Spread tomato, basil, and capers evenly over pizza crust.

3. Sprinkle the cheese on top and bake on rack in the oven for 15 minutes.

Exchanges/Choices
1 Starch
1/2 Fat

Calories	110
Calories from Fat	20
Total Fat	2.5 g
Saturated Fat	1.4 g
Trans Fat	0 g
Cholesterol	0 mg
Sodium	295 mg
Total Carbohydrate	18 g
Dietary Fiber	3 g
Sugars	2 g
Protein	6 g

Cooking Tip:
Quick, healthy, and full of flavor, this pizza will be a hit. Serve it with a green salad for a side.

MEXICAN LASAGNA

Serves 12 • Serving Size: 1 slice • Prep Time: 20 minutes

Cooking spray

1 lb lean ground turkey breast

1 16-oz can fat-free refried beans

1 8-oz can no-salt-added tomato sauce

1/4 cup salsa

1 Tbsp chili powder

1 tsp garlic powder

1 4-oz can mild green chilies, chopped

8 whole-wheat tortillas*

1 1/2 cups reduced-fat, shredded Mexican cheese

1 medium tomato, diced

1. Preheat oven to 350°F. Coat a large glass or metal baking dish with cooking spray.

2. In a large nonstick skillet, cook ground turkey for 7–9 minutes or until it begins to brown. Drain excess fat. Stir in refried beans, tomato sauce, salsa, chili powder, garlic powder, and green chilies. Reduce heat and cook for 3 minutes.

3. Cover bottom of baking dish with four tortillas. Spoon half of turkey mixture over the tortillas. Top with four more tortillas and remaining turkey mixture. Sprinkle cheese on top.

4. Bake for 25 minutes. Top with diced tomatoes.

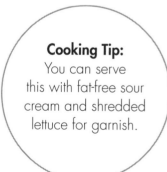

Cooking Tip:
You can serve this with fat-free sour cream and shredded lettuce for garnish.

*Each tortilla should have 30 g carbohydrate and 4 g dietary fiber per serving.

Exchanges/Choices
1 1/2 Starch
1 Vegetable
2 Lean Meat

Calories 235
   Calories from Fat.....55
Total Fat ....6 g
   Saturated Fat ....1.8 g
   Trans Fat ....0 g
Cholesterol ....35 mg
Sodium ....610 mg
Total Carbohydrate....27 g
   Dietary Fiber ....6 g
   Sugars ....3 g
Protein ....18 g

MEXICAN SOUP

Serves 8 • Serving Size: 1 cup • Prep Time: 20 minutes

2 whole-wheat tortillas, cut into strips*

Cooking spray

2 4-oz boneless, skinless chicken breasts, cut into 1-inch strips

1/2 tsp garlic powder

1/4 tsp ground black pepper

1/2 medium onion, diced

1 large tomato, diced

48 oz reduced-sodium, fat-free chicken broth

2 tsp fresh cilantro, minced

1 tsp dried oregano

1/2 tsp cumin

1/2 lime, juiced

1 15-oz can black beans, rinsed and drained

1 cup frozen corn kernels

1. Preheat oven to 400°F. Spray tortillas with cooking spray and place on baking sheet. Bake for 10 minutes, until crisp.

2. In a large pot coated with cooking spray, add the chicken over high heat and cook until light brown. Sprinkle with garlic powder and pepper. Add onions and tomato; sauté for 2 minutes.

3. Add broth, cilantro, oregano, cumin, and lime juice. Bring to a boil, then reduce heat and simmer for 10 minutes.

4. Add beans and corn; cook for 5 minutes.

5. Ladle soup into bowls and top with tortilla strips.

Cooking Tip:
Top each bowl of soup with two avocado slices, if desired.

Exchanges/Choices
1 1/2 Starch
1 Lean Meat

Calories 150
    Calories from Fat..... 20
Total Fat .... 2 g
    Saturated Fat .... 0.3 g
    Trans Fat .... 0 g
Cholesterol .... 15 mg
Sodium .... 530 mg
Total Carbohydrate .... 21 g
    Dietary Fiber .... 5 g
    Sugars .... 3 g
Protein .... 12 g

*Each tortilla should have 30 g carbohydrate and 4 g dietary fiber per serving.

MOO SHOO CHICKEN

Serves 5 • Serving Size: 2 tortillas • Prep Time: 5 minutes

1 Tbsp canola oil

5 green onions, chopped

3 cups prepackaged coleslaw mix

1 cup shredded carrots

2 cups cooked chicken, shredded (about 1 large breast)

1/4 cup plum sauce

1/4 cup reduced-sodium, fat-free chicken broth

10 whole-wheat tortillas (about 6 inches in diameter each)

1. Add oil to a large skillet over medium-high heat. Add green onions, coleslaw mix, and carrots. Stir-fry for 3–4 minutes or until cabbage begins to wilt but is still a little crunchy.

2. Add chicken, plum sauce, and chicken broth. Bring to a simmer for 2 minutes.

3. Heat tortillas in the microwave and divide the moo shoo chicken evenly among the 10 tortillas.

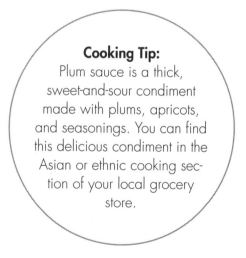

Cooking Tip:
Plum sauce is a thick, sweet-and-sour condiment made with plums, apricots, and seasonings. You can find this delicious condiment in the Asian or ethnic cooking section of your local grocery store.

Exchanges/Choices
2 Starch
1 Vegetable
2 Lean Meat
1 Fat

Calories 340
   Calories from Fat.....80
Total Fat ....9 g
   Saturated Fat............1.1 g
   Trans Fat ....0 g
Cholesterol ....50 mg
Sodium ....655 mg
Total Carbohydrate ....41 g
   Dietary Fiber ....6 g
   Sugars ....10 g
Protein ....22 g

MUSHROOM-STUFFED TURKEY BREAST

Serves 4 • Serving Size: 1 turkey breast • Prep Time: 15 minutes

1 Tbsp canola oil

4 oz assorted wild mushrooms, finely chopped

2 Tbsp fresh chives, chopped

1/2 tsp garlic powder

1 1/4 lb turkey breast, cut into 4-oz portions, pounded to 1/2 inch thick

Cooking spray

1/2 tsp salt (*optional*)

1/4 tsp ground black pepper

2 Tbsp light mayonnaise

2 Tbsp grated Parmesan cheese

1. Preheat oven to 375°F.

2. Add canola oil to a sauté pan over medium-high heat. Add mushrooms and sauté for 5–7 minutes or until all liquid is evaporated. Set aside to cool.

3. In a medium bowl, combine mushrooms, chives, and garlic powder. Lay pounded turkey breasts on a clean cutting board. Spoon 1/4 of mushroom mixture on each breast and spread evenly to about 1/4 inch from the sides. Fold over each breast and secure with a toothpick.

4. Coat a baking sheet with cooking spray. Lay each breast down on the sheet. Season with salt (optional) and ground black pepper. Spread 1/2 Tbsp of mayonnaise on each breast and sprinkle with 1/2 Tbsp of Parmesan cheese. Lightly spray each breast with cooking spray.

5. Bake for 25 minutes or until juices run clear. Remove toothpick before serving.

Exchanges/Choices
5 Lean Meat

Calories	225
Calories from Fat	70
Total Fat	8 g
Saturated Fat	1.4 g
Trans Fat	0 g
Cholesterol	95 mg
Sodium	140 mg
Total Carbohydrate	2 g
Dietary Fiber	0 g
Sugars	1 g
Protein	36 g

Cooking Tip:
Wild mushrooms are often prepackaged in the grocery store. If you can't find them, try crimini (or baby portobellos) mixed with regular button mushrooms.

MUSHROOM TURKEY BURGERS WITH BLEU CHEESE

Serves 6 • Serving Size: 1 burger • Prep Time: 10 minutes

Cooking spray

1 cup mushrooms, minced

1 1/4 lb lean ground turkey breast

1/2 tsp onion powder

1/2 tsp garlic powder

1/2 tsp ground black pepper

2 oz bleu cheese, crumbled

6 large tomato slices

6 small whole-wheat hamburger buns

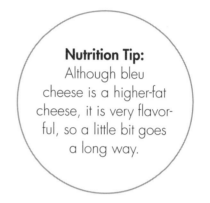

Nutrition Tip:
Although bleu cheese is a higher-fat cheese, it is very flavorful, so a little bit goes a long way.

1. Prepare an indoor or outdoor grill.

2. Coat a nonstick skillet with cooking spray over medium-high heat. Add mushrooms and cook until no liquid remains, about 5–7 minutes. Set aside to cool.

3. In a medium bowl, combine all ingredients (except tomato and buns) with cooled mushrooms. Divide turkey into six equal portions, shaping each into a 1/2-inch thick patty.

4. Place patties on grill rack; grill 7 minutes on each side or until done (or coat a large skillet with nonstick cooking spray and cook patties over medium heat for 3–4 minutes per side, or until juices run clear).

5. Serve burgers with a tomato slice on whole-wheat hamburger buns.

Exchanges/Choices
1 1/2 Starch
3 Lean Meat

Calories 260
   Calories from Fat.....45
Total Fat ....5 g
   Saturated Fat ....2.2 g
   Trans Fat ....0 g
Cholesterol ....70 mg
Sodium ....380 mg
Total Carbohydrate ....24 g
   Dietary Fiber ....4 g
   Sugars ....5 g
Protein ....29 g

MUSTARD-GLAZED SALMON WITH GREEN BEANS

Serves 4 • Serving Size: 1 packet • Prep Time: 10 minutes

4 sheets (12 × 19 inches) aluminum foil

Cooking spray

1 Tbsp Splenda Brown Sugar Blend

1 Tbsp trans-fat-free margarine

1/4 cup Dijon mustard

1 Tbsp lite soy sauce

4 cups frozen green beans, thawed

4 4-oz salmon fillets

Cooking Tip:
If you want to use the oven instead, preheat the oven to 400°F and bake these packets on a baking sheet for 20 minutes.

1. Prepare an outdoor grill (see cooking tip). Spray aluminum foil with cooking spray.

2. In a small bowl, mix together Splenda Brown Sugar Blend, margarine, mustard, and soy sauce.

3. Place 1 cup green beans on each sheet of foil. Place salmon fillet on top of green beans. Top salmon with 1/4 Brown Sugar Blend mixture, spread evenly over salmon.

4. Bring up sides of foil. Double fold top and ends to seal packet, leaving a little room in packet for circulation. Repeat for remaining three packets.

5. Place packets in covered outdoor grill on medium-high heat and cook for 12–14 minutes, until salmon flakes with fork.

Exchanges/Choices
2 Vegetable
3 Lean Meat
2 Fat

Calories	280
Calories from Fat	115
Total Fat	13 g
Saturated Fat	2.4 g
Trans Fat	0 g
Cholesterol	75 mg
Sodium	595 mg
Total Carbohydrate	15 g
Dietary Fiber	5 g
Sugars	8 g
Protein	27 g

ONE-POT SKILLET

Serves 7 • Serving Size: 1 cup • Prep Time: 5 minutes

2 cups whole-wheat rotini pasta, uncooked

1 lb lean ground turkey breast

1 medium onion, diced

1 14.5-oz can no-salt-added crushed tomatoes

1 8-oz can tomato sauce

2 tsp chili powder

1/8 tsp cayenne pepper (*optional*)

1 tsp garlic powder

1 tsp Splenda

1 cup reduced-fat, shredded Monterey Jack cheese

1. Cook pasta according to package directions, omitting salt. Drain.

2. In a large skillet, cook ground turkey until it begins to brown, about 6–7 minutes. Drain excess fat. Add onions and sauté about 5 more minutes or until translucent.

3. Add next six ingredients and bring to a boil. Reduce heat and simmer for 6–7 minutes or until it begins to thicken. Fold in cheese and toss with drained pasta.

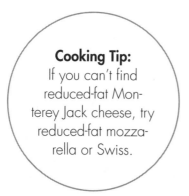

Cooking Tip:
If you can't find reduced-fat Monterey Jack cheese, try reduced-fat mozzarella or Swiss.

Exchanges/Choices
1 Starch
2 Vegetable
2 Lean Meat

Calories 225	
Calories from Fat.....40	
Total Fat ....4.5 g	
Saturated Fat ....2.2 g	
Trans Fat ....0 g	
Cholesterol ....55 mg	
Sodium ....390 mg	
Total Carbohydrate ....25 g	
Dietary Fiber ....4 g	
Sugars ....5 g	
Protein ....23 g	

OPEN-FACED BARBEQUED PORK SANDWICH

Serves 4 • Serving Size: 1 sandwich • Prep Time: 10 minutes

Cooking spray
1 1-lb pork tenderloin
1/4 tsp ground black pepper
1 tsp dried thyme
2/3 cup barbeque sauce
2 whole-wheat hamburger buns

1. Preheat oven to 375°F. Coat a baking sheet with cooking spray.

2. Season pork tenderloin on all sides with black pepper and thyme. Place on baking sheet and roast in the oven for 40 minutes. Remove from oven and let sit for 10–15 minutes.

3. Slice pork tenderloin thinly. Add barbeque sauce to a medium saucepan and heat over medium heat. Stir in sliced pork.

4. Toast hamburger buns. Open buns and top each with 1/4 of sliced pork.

Exchanges/Choices
1 Starch
1 Carbohydrate
3 Lean Meat

Calories	265
Calories from Fat	35
Total Fat	4 g
Saturated Fat	1.2 g
Trans Fat	0 g
Cholesterol	60 mg
Sodium	510 mg
Total Carbohydrate	33 g
Dietary Fiber	2 g
Sugars	22 g
Protein	24 g

Cooking Tip:
Top these tangy sandwiches with sliced onion and pickles for some crunch.

This recipe is high in sodium.

ORANGE ROUGHY PACKET WITH SUMMER SQUASH

Serves 4 • Serving Size: 1 packet • Prep Time: 10 minutes

4 sheets (12 × 19 inches) aluminum foil

Cooking spray

2 medium yellow squash, thinly sliced
    into rounds

4 4-oz orange roughy fillets

1/2 tsp salt (*optional*)

1/2 tsp ground black pepper

1 cup nonfat, plain yogurt

2 Tbsp chopped fresh chives

Cooking Tip:
These packets can be done on an outdoor grill if you don't want to use your oven. Just place them directly on the grill rack, put the lid on, and cook for 15 minutes.

1. Preheat oven to 450°F (see tip).

2. Spray aluminum foil with cooking spray.

3. Divide the yellow squash slices evenly among the four pieces of foil. Top each with one orange roughy fillet. Season with salt (optional) and pepper.

4. In a small bowl, whisk together yogurt and chives. Divide evenly over four fillets.

5. Bring up sides of foil. Double fold top and ends to seal packet, leaving a little room in packet for circulation. Repeat for remaining three packets.

6. Place packets on a baking sheet and bake for 12–15 minutes.

Exchanges/Choices
1/2 Carbohydrate
3 Lean Meat

Calories 140
   Calories from Fat 10
Total Fat .... 1 g
   Saturated Fat .... 0.1 g
   Trans Fat .... 0 g
Cholesterol .... 75 mg
Sodium .... 105 mg
Total Carbohydrate ...... 8 g
   Dietary Fiber .... 1 g
   Sugars .... 6 g
Protein .... 24 g

OVEN-FRIED CHICKEN

Serves 4 • Serving Size: 1 chicken breast • Prep Time: 15 minutes

Cooking spray

1 1/2 cups bran flake crumbs

1 tsp paprika

1/2 tsp dried thyme

1/2 tsp garlic powder

1/2 tsp onion powder

1 egg

2 egg whites

1 tsp hot sauce (*optional*)

2 Tbsp whole-wheat flour

4 4-oz boneless, skinless chicken breasts

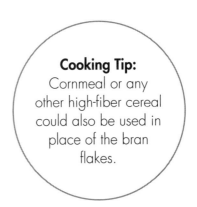

Cooking Tip:
Cornmeal or any other high-fiber cereal could also be used in place of the bran flakes.

1. Preheat oven to 350°F. Coat a shallow baking pan with cooking spray.

2. In a medium bowl, combine bran flake crumbs, paprika, thyme, garlic powder, and onion powder.

3. In a separate bowl, lightly beat egg and egg whites. Add hot sauce and mix well.

4. In a separate bowl add flour.

5. Dip each chicken breast in the flour, then egg mixture, and then in branflake mixture. Coat each side of chicken breast.

6. Place chicken breasts in a baking pan. Spray chicken lightly with cooking spray and bake 30–35 minutes, until juice run clear.

Exchanges/Choices
1 1/2 Starch
3 Lean Meat

Calories 220
  Calories from Fat 35
Total Fat .... 4 g
  Saturated Fat .... 1 g
  Trans Fat .... 0 g
Cholesterol .... 100 mg
Sodium .... 330 mg
Total Carbohydrate .... 25 g
  Dietary Fiber .... 6 g
  Sugars .... 4 g
Protein .... 24 g

PESTO PASTA WITH SHRIMP

Serves 5 • Serving Size: 1/5th recipe • Prep Time: 5 minutes

4 oz whole-wheat angel hair pasta, uncooked

1 lb cooked shrimp

4 Tbsp jarred pesto sauce

1. Cook pasta according to package directions, omitting salt; drain.

2. Add cooked shrimp to pasta pot and heat through. Add drained pasta and pesto sauce to pot with shrimp; toss to coat pasta with sauce.

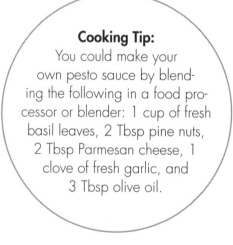

Cooking Tip:
You could make your own pesto sauce by blending the following in a food processor or blender: 1 cup of fresh basil leaves, 2 Tbsp pine nuts, 2 Tbsp Parmesan cheese, 1 clove of fresh garlic, and 3 Tbsp olive oil.

Exchanges/Choices
1 Starch
3 Lean Meat
1 Fat

Calories 255
   Calories from Fat.....80
Total Fat ....9 g
   Saturated Fat ....1.5 g
   Trans Fat ....0 g
Cholesterol ....175 mg
Sodium ....305 mg
Total Carbohydrate ....19 g
   Dietary Fiber ....1 g
   Sugars ....2 g
Protein ....23 g

PINEAPPLE PISTACHIO PORK CHOPS

Serves 4 • Serving Size: 1 pork chop • Prep Time: 10 minutes

4 boneless pork loin chops (about 4 oz each)

1/4 tsp garlic salt

1/2 tsp ground black pepper

1 tsp olive oil

Cooking spray

1 8-oz can crushed pineapple in juice, drained

2 Tbsp balsamic vinegar

3 Tbsp hulled pistachios, chopped and toasted

1. Season pork chops well with garlic salt and pepper.

2. Add oil to a large nonstick skillet over medium-high heat. Sauté chops for 6–8 minutes or until nicely browned, turning once. Remove from pan; keep warm.

3. Spray pan with cooking spray. Add pineapple and balsamic vinegar and simmer for 5–7 minutes or until sauce takes on a glaze-like consistency.

4. Pour pineapple sauce over pork chops. Top with pistachios.

Exchanges/Choices
1/2 Fruit
3 Lean Meat
1 1/2 Fat

Calories 225
  Calories from Fat...100
Total Fat ....11 g
  Saturated Fat ....3 g
  Trans Fat ....0 g
Cholesterol ....60 mg
Sodium ....125 mg
Total Carbohydrate ......9 g
  Dietary Fiber ....1 g
  Sugars ....7 g
Protein ....22 g

Cooking Tip:
Don't overcook the pork! Overcooking makes pork tough and chewy.

PISTACHIO CRUSTED SALMON

Serves 4 • Serving Size: 1 fillet • Prep Time: 5 minutes

6 Tbsp hulled pistachios, finely chopped
1/4 cup buckwheat flour
2 egg whites, beaten
4 4-oz salmon fillets
Cooking spray

1. Preheat oven to 400°F.

2. In a shallow dish, combine pistachios and flour. In another shallow dish, add egg whites.

3. Dip one side of the salmon in egg whites and then press into pistachio mixture.

4. Place fillets nut side up on nonstick baking sheet.

5. Repeat for remaining three fillets. Spray top of fillets with cooking spray.

6. Bake for 25 minutes.

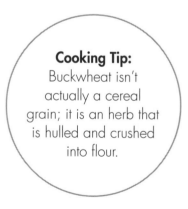

Cooking Tip:
Buckwheat isn't actually a cereal grain; it is an herb that is hulled and crushed into flour.

Exchanges/Choices
1/2 Starch
4 Lean Meat
1 1/2 Fat

Calories 295
    Calories from Fat...135
Total Fat ....15 g
    Saturated Fat ....2.4 g
    Trans Fat ....0 g
Cholesterol ....75 mg
Sodium ....85 mg
Total Carbohydrate ......9 g
    Dietary Fiber ....2 g
    Sugars ....1 g
Protein ....29 g

the healthy carb diabetes cookbook

PORK TENDERLOIN WITH PEACH MANGO SALSA

Serves 4 • Serving Size: 1/4th recipe • Prep Time: 35 minutes

2 tsp dried oregano

1 tsp cumin

1/4 tsp ground black pepper

1 tsp garlic powder

1 lime, juiced

1 lb pork tenderloin

1/2 cup jarred peach mango salsa (see tip)

1. Preheat oven to 375°F.

2. In a small bowl, combine spices and rub over the whole pork tenderloin. Place pork in baking dish and pour lime juice over it. Marinate pork for 30 minutes in the refrigerator.

3. Pour salsa over pork and bake 40 minutes or until done.

Exchanges/Choices
1/2 Carbohydrate
3 Lean Meat

Calories	140
Calories from Fat	25
Total Fat	3 g
Saturated Fat	1 g
Trans Fat	0 g
Cholesterol	60 mg
Sodium	195 mg
Total Carbohydrate	6 g
Dietary Fiber	0 g
Sugars	3 g
Protein	22 g

Cooking Tip:
If you can't find peach mango salsa, you can substitute any fruit-based salsa, such as pineapple.

PUMPKIN SOUP

Serves 12 • Serving Size: 1 cup • Prep Time: 45 minutes

1 tsp olive oil

Cooking spray

2 celery stalks, diced small

1 medium onion, diced small

48 oz reduced-sodium, fat-free chicken broth

Pinch ground nutmeg

1 tsp dried sage

1/2 tsp salt (*optional*)

1/4 tsp ground black pepper

2 15-oz cans pure pumpkin

1 cup fat-free half-and-half, heated

Lime Cream

1/2 cup reduced-fat sour cream

Juice of 1 small lime

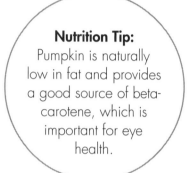

Nutrition Tip:
Pumpkin is naturally low in fat and provides a good source of beta-carotene, which is important for eye health.

1. Add oil and a generous amount of cooking spray to a large soup pot. Sauté celery and onion over medium-high heat for 5–6 minutes or until onion is clear.

2. Add chicken broth, nutmeg, sage, salt (optional), and pepper and bring to a boil. Reduce heat and simmer for 15 minutes.

3. Add pumpkin and simmer for an additional 15 minutes.

4. Stir in heated half-and-half. Working in batches, puree soup in a blender until smooth. (You can also use an immersion blender right in the soup pot to puree soup.)

5. In a small bowl, mix together sour cream and lime juice. Serve soup topped with a spoonful of lime cream.

Exchanges/Choices
1/2 Carbohydrate
1/2 Fat

Calories	65
Calories from Fat	15
Total Fat	1.5 g
Saturated Fat	1 g
Trans Fat	0 g
Cholesterol	5 mg
Sodium	275 mg
Total Carbohydrate	10 g
Dietary Fiber	2 g
Sugars	5 g
Protein	3 g

RED ONION STEAK

Serves 4 • Serving Size: 1 steak • Prep Time: 10 minutes

1 1/2 Tbsp olive oil, divided

1 small red onion, sliced

2 Tbsp sugar-free apricot preserves

2 Tbsp balsamic vinegar

1/3 cup reduced-sodium, fat-free chicken broth

1 lb beef tenderloin (4 4-oz steaks)

1/2 tsp salt (*optional*)

1/2 tsp ground black pepper

1. Add 2 tsp olive oil to a large sauté pan over medium-high heat. Add onion and sauté until it begins to caramelize.

2. Add apricot preserves, vinegar, and chicken broth and bring to a simmer. Cook until liquid is reduced by half.

3. Season both sides of the steaks with salt (optional) and pepper. Add remaining oil to a large sauté pan and sear steaks on both sides on high heat for 3–4 minutes or until cooked to medium well.

4. Divide red onion sauce evenly among the four steaks.

Exchanges/Choices
1/2 Carbohydrate
3 Lean Meat
1 Fat

Calories	210
Calories from Fat	100
Total Fat	11 g
Saturated Fat	2.9 g
Trans Fat	0 g
Cholesterol	60 mg
Sodium	85 mg
Total Carbohydrate	6 g
Dietary Fiber	0 g
Sugars	2 g
Protein	21 g

Nutrition Tip:
You can also grill this steak for even lower-fat cooking. Grilling allows the fat to drip from the meat, resulting in a leaner food.

ROASTED EGGPLANT CRUSTED SALMON

Serves 4 • Serving Size: 1 fillet • Prep Time: 30 minutes

1/2 Tbsp olive oil

1 small eggplant, peeled and diced

2 garlic cloves, minced

4 4-oz skinless salmon fillets

1/2 tsp salt (*optional*)

1/4 tsp ground black pepper

Cooking spray

2 Tbsp grated Parmesan cheese

Nutrition Tip:
The American Heart Association recommends eating fish two times per week, especially those with omega-3 fatty acids, such as tuna, salmon, and herring.

1. Preheat oven to 375°F.

2. In a medium bowl, toss together olive oil, eggplant, and garlic.

3. Spread mixture on a baking sheet and bake for 20–25 minutes or until eggplant begins to brown.

4. Add roasted eggplant to a food processor or blender and puree until smooth.

5. Season each side of the four salmon fillets with salt (optional) and pepper.

6. Coat a baking sheet with cooking spray. Place salmon fillets on baking sheet and divide the eggplant mixture evenly among each fillet. Spread the eggplant mixture over each fillet, so the top of each fillet is covered with eggplant.

7. Sprinkle the Parmesan cheese over each fillet and bake for 15 minutes or until salmon flakes with a fork.

Exchanges/Choices
2 Vegetable
3 Lean Meat
1 1/2 Fat

Calories	255
Calories from Fat	115
Total Fat	13 g
Saturated Fat	2.5 g
Trans Fat	0 g
Cholesterol	80 mg
Sodium	80 mg
Total Carbohydrate	10 g
Dietary Fiber	3 g
Sugars	3 g
Protein	26 g

the healthy carb diabetes cookbook

ROASTED GARLIC ORANGE ROUGHY

Serves 4 • Serving Size: 1 fillet • Prep Time: 40 minutes

Cooking spray

Garlic head

1 1/2 tsp olive oil (reserve 1 tsp)

4 4-oz orange roughy fillets

3 Tbsp grated Parmesan cheese

Dash paprika

1/4 tsp ground black pepper

1/2 tsp salt (*optional*)

Cooking Tip:
A head of garlic looks like a bulb and is made up of many sections called cloves. Roasting the cloves in the casing ensures maximum flavor!

1. Preheat oven to 375°F. Coat a baking dish with cooking spray.

2. Cut the top off a whole head of garlic. Place cut side up on a medium piece of foil. Drizzle 1/2 tsp olive oil on the garlic head. Fold foil up on all sides; seal. Bake on the oven rack for 40 minutes.

3. Remove garlic from foil and squeeze roasted garlic cloves out of husk into a small bowl. Add 1 tsp olive oil and blend well.

4. Place fish on baking sheet coated with cooking spray. Spread roasted garlic evenly over each fillet. Sprinkle each fillet evenly with Parmesan cheese and season with paprika, pepper, and salt (optional).

5. Bake for 20 minutes.

Exchanges/Choices
1 Vegetable
4 Lean Meat

Calories	190
Calories from Fat	45
Total Fat	5 g
Saturated Fat	1.4 g
Trans Fat	0 g
Cholesterol	100 mg
Sodium	130 mg
Total Carbohydrate	5 g
Dietary Fiber	0 g
Sugars	0 g
Protein	30 g

ROASTED ITALIAN VEGETABLE AND SAUSAGE PASTA

Serves 11 • Serving Size: 1 1/2 cups • Prep Time: 25 minutes

1 lb whole-wheat penne pasta, uncooked

5 Italian turkey sausage links, cut into 1-inch pieces

Cooking spray

1 Tbsp olive oil

1 eggplant, cut into 1-inch cubes

2 zucchini, cut into 1-inch cubes

5 plum (roma) tomatoes, cut into 1-inch cubes

1 green pepper, cut into 1-inch pieces

4 cloves garlic, crushed

1/4 tsp salt (*optional*)

1/4 tsp ground black pepper

3 Tbsp grated Parmesan cheese

Cooking Tip:
Al dente translates as "to the tooth." This means that your pasta or veggies are cooked through, but not mushy; they still have a little bite.

1. Cook pasta according to package directions, omitting salt. Drain.

2. In a deep sauté pan over medium-high heat, cook sausage for 10 minutes or until done. Remove from pan.

3. Spray pan with cooking spray and add olive oil and remaining ingredients except cheese and pasta. Sauté for 20 minutes or until vegetables are al dente.

4. Add sausage back to vegetables and sauté for 2–3 minutes.

5. In a large bowl, toss together pasta with vegetable mixture. Sprinkle with Parmesan cheese and serve immediately.

Exchanges/Choices
2 Starch
2 Vegetable
1 Fat

Calories	260
Calories from Fat	65
Total Fat	7 g
Saturated Fat	1.7 g
Trans Fat	0 g
Cholesterol	30 mg
Sodium	245 mg
Total Carbohydrate	39 g
Dietary Fiber	7 g
Sugars	5 g
Protein	14 g

the healthy carb diabetes cookbook

ROASTED TOMATO AND BASIL CHICKEN

Serves 4 • Serving Size: 1/4th recipe • Prep Time: 10 minutes

1 Tbsp olive oil

Cooking spray

1/2 tsp garlic powder

1/4 tsp ground black pepper

1 lb boneless, skinless chicken breasts

5 plum (roma) tomatoes, quartered

3 garlic cloves, minced

1/4 cup fresh basil, chopped

1. Preheat oven to 375°F.

2. Add olive oil to a large oven-safe skillet coated with cooking spray. Season the chicken with garlic powder and ground black pepper. Add chicken to pan and sear on high heat for 3 minutes on each side.

3. Add tomatoes and garlic to pan on top of chicken breasts and toss. Place skillet in oven and bake for 25 minutes.

4. Remove from oven and top with basil.

Exchanges/Choices
1 Vegetable
3 Lean Meat
1/2 Fat

Calories	185
Calories from Fat	55
Total Fat	6 g
Saturated Fat	1.3 g
Trans Fat	0 g
Cholesterol	65 mg
Sodium	65 mg
Total Carbohydrate	6 g
Dietary Fiber	2 g
Sugars	4 g
Protein	25 g

Cooking Tip:
This recipe can be eaten alone or served over whole-wheat pasta.

SAUERKRAUT AND SAUSAGE SKILLET

Serves 6 • Serving Size: 1/6th recipe • Prep Time: 5 minutes

Cooking spray

1 lb lean turkey or low-fat kielbasa, cut into 1-inch chunks

1 32-oz jar sauerkraut, drained

2 Tbsp Splenda Brown Sugar Blend

1 Tbsp cider vinegar

1 cup cooked brown rice

1. Coat a large, deep skillet with cooking spray. Over medium-high heat, sauté sausage until lightly browned. Remove from pan.

2. Coat pan with cooking spray again. Add sauerkraut to pan and sauté for 3–4 minutes. Add Splenda Brown Sugar Blend and vinegar; sauté an additional 3 minutes.

3. Add sausage and brown rice to pan, heat through.

Cooking Tip:
Making one-pot meals saves time during cooking and cleanup.

Exchanges/Choices	
1/2 Starch	
1/2 Carbohydrate	
1 Vegetable	
2 Lean Meat	

Calories	175
Calories from Fat	40
Total Fat	4.5 g
Saturated Fat	1.4 g
Trans Fat	0 g
Cholesterol	45 mg
Sodium	1345 mg
Total Carbohydrate	19 g
Dietary Fiber	4 g
Sugars	8 g
Protein	14 g

This recipe is high in sodium.

SAUSAGE LASAGNA

Serves 10 • Serving Size: 1 slice • Prep Time: 15 minutes

Cooking spray

12 strips whole-wheat lasagna noodles

1 lb turkey Italian sausage

1 2-lb, 13-oz jar pasta sauce

1 1/2 cups reduced-fat, shredded mozzarella cheese, divided

15 oz fat-free ricotta cheese

1/4 cup grated Parmesan cheese

1 egg, slightly beaten

1/4 cup fresh parsley, chopped

1. Preheat oven to 350°F. Spray a 13 × 9 × 2-inch glass baking dish with cooking spray.

2. Cook noodles according to package directions, omitting salt.

3. Cut ends of turkey sausage and squeeze sausage meat out of the casings. Discard casings.

4. In a large saucepan, cook turkey sausage over medium-high heat until brown. Drain fat. Lower heat to medium and add pasta sauce. Cook for 5 minutes. Set aside to cool.

Cooking Tip:
Feel free to add any veggies, such as mushrooms, green pepper, and zucchini, to the pasta sauce, if desired.

5. In a medium bowl, mix together 1/2 cup mozzarella (reserve 1 cup mozzarella), ricotta cheese, Parmesan cheese, egg, and parsley.

6. Spread 1 cup pasta sauce and sausage on bottom of baking dish. Arrange noodles side by side on top of sauce. Spread 1/3 of the cheese mixture on top of noodles.

7. Repeat layering with pasta sauce, noodles, and cheese mixtures two more times.

8. Top with remaining 3 noodles and 1 cup of sauce. Cover lasagna with foil and bake 25 minutes. Uncover; top with remaining mozzarella cheese and bake additional 25 minutes or until cheese is lightly golden brown.

This recipe is high in sodium.

Exchanges/Choices
2 1/2 Starch
2 Lean Meat
1/2 Fat

Calories	305
Calories from Fat	65
Total Fat	7 g
Saturated Fat	3 g
Trans Fat	0 g
Cholesterol	70 mg
Sodium	770 mg
Total Carbohydrate	36 g
Dietary Fiber	4 g
Sugars	11 g
Protein	23 g

SHRIMP FAJITAS

Serves 5 • Serving Size: 2 fajitas • Prep Time: 15 minutes

Cooking spray

1 lb medium shrimp, peeled and deveined

1 tsp canola oil

2 green bell peppers, sliced into thin strips

1 medium onion, sliced into thin strips

1/4 cup water

1/2 Tbsp chili powder

1/4 tsp cayenne pepper (*optional*)

1/4 tsp cumin

1/2 tsp salt (*optional*)

1/2 tsp ground black pepper

10 6-inch whole-wheat tortillas

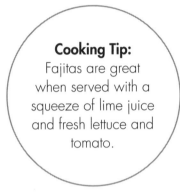

Cooking Tip:
Fajitas are great when served with a squeeze of lime juice and fresh lettuce and tomato.

1. Coat a large nonstick skillet with cooking spray. Cook shrimp over medium heat for about 2 minutes. Remove from pan and set aside.

2. Add oil to the pan and heat. Add peppers and onion; cook about 7 minutes or until they begin to brown. Add shrimp and any juices back to pan.

3. Add water and spices, including salt (optional) and pepper. Bring to a boil; reduce heat and simmer until water evaporates. Serve with tortillas.

Exchanges/Choices
2 Starch
1 Vegetable
1 Lean Meat
1/2 Fat

Calories	255
Calories from Fat	45
Total Fat	5 g
Saturated Fat	0.5 g
Trans Fat	0 g
Cholesterol	105 mg
Sodium	520 mg
Total Carbohydrate	34 g
Dietary Fiber	6 g
Sugars	4 g
Protein	16 g

SHRIMP SCAMPI PASTA

Serves 8 • Serving Size: 1 cup • Prep Time: 5 minutes

1/2 lb whole-wheat penne pasta

2 Tbsp olive oil

1 1/2 lb shrimp, peeled and deveined

5 cloves garlic, minced

1/2 tsp crushed red pepper flakes

1/2 cup pasta water

1/4 tsp ground black pepper

1. Cook pasta according to package directions, omitting salt. Drain; reserve 1/2 cup pasta water.

2. Add olive oil to a large skillet over medium heat. Sauté shrimp, garlic, and red pepper flakes in olive oil until shrimp are pink and slightly firm, about 3–4 minutes.

3. Add reserved pasta water, black pepper, and pasta.

4. Toss to coat.

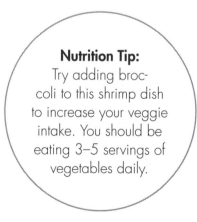

Nutrition Tip:
Try adding broccoli to this shrimp dish to increase your veggie intake. You should be eating 3–5 servings of vegetables daily.

Exchanges/Choices
1 1/2 Starch
1 Lean Meat
1/2 Fat

Calories	180
Calories from Fat	40
Total Fat	4.5 g
Saturated Fat	0.7 g
Trans Fat	0 g
Cholesterol	100 mg
Sodium	115 mg
Total Carbohydrate	22 g
Dietary Fiber	3 g
Sugars	1 g
Protein	14 g

SPICY TURKEY BURGER

Serves 6 • Serving Size: 1 burger • Prep Time: 10 minutes

1 1/4 lb lean ground turkey breast

1/2 cup salsa

1 egg white

1 clove garlic, minced

1/2 tsp Mrs. Dash seasoning

6 whole-wheat hamburger buns

Sauce

4 Tbsp light ranch dressing

1 tsp hot sauce

1. Prepare an indoor or outdoor grill.

2. In a large bowl, combine ground turkey, salsa, egg white, garlic, and Mrs. Dash. Mix well. Divide into six equal portions and form into 1/2-inch thick patties.

3. Place patties on grill rack and grill for 7 minutes on each side until done (or coat a large nonstick skillet with cooking spray and cook patties over medium heat for 3–4 minutes per side, until juices run clear).

4. In a small bowl, combine ranch dressing and hot sauce.

5. Place one patty and approximately 2 tsp ranch mixture on a whole-wheat bun. Repeat for remaining five burgers.

Exchanges/Choices
1 1/2 Starch
3 Lean Meat

Calories	250
Calories from Fat	45
Total Fat	5 g
Saturated Fat	0.7 g
Trans Fat	0 g
Cholesterol	65 mg
Sodium	490 mg
Total Carbohydrate	25 g
Dietary Fiber	4 g
Sugars	5 g
Protein	27 g

Nutrition Tip:
If you like a milder flavor, use a mild or medium salsa and half the amount of hot sauce. You'll get the same great flavor, just a little less kick!

This recipe is high in sodium.

SPINACH TORTELLINI WITH SALAD

Serves 4 • Serving Size: 1 cup • Prep Time: 30 minutes

Tortellini

1 9-oz pkg whole-wheat cheese tortellini, uncooked

Cooking spray

9 oz frozen, chopped spinach, thawed and drained

2 Tbsp trans-fat-free margarine

2 Tbsp grated Parmesan cheese

2 Tbsp fresh basil, chopped

2 Tbsp fresh oregano, chopped

1/2 cup pasta water

Salad

8 cups salad greens mix

4 tomato slices

1/2 cup diced cucumber

1/4 cup fat-free Italian salad dressing

1. Cook tortellini according to package directions, omitting salt. Drain and reserve 1/2 cup pasta water.

2. Coat a medium sauté pan with cooking spray. Add spinach to pan and heat over medium-high heat for approximately 5 minutes. Remove spinach from pan.

3. Combine margarine, Parmesan cheese, basil, and oregano, and add to pan over low heat. Melt slowly and stir.

4. Place tortellini in the sauté pan with the melted butter and herbs. Add the spinach and the reserved pasta water; toss to combine. Cook for about 30 seconds.

5. Prepare the four side salads (2 cups salad greens, 1 tomato slice, 2 Tbsp diced cucumbers, and 1 Tbsp salad dressing).

Cooking Tip:
You can find the whole-wheat tortellini in the refrigerated pasta section at your local grocery store.

Exchanges/Choices
2 Starch
1 Vegetable
1 Lean Meat
1 1/2 Fat

Calories	285
Calories from Fat	100
Total Fat	11 g
Saturated Fat	3.4 g
Trans Fat	0 g
Cholesterol	40 mg
Sodium	575 mg
Total Carbohydrate	35 g
Dietary Fiber	8 g
Sugars	6 g
Protein	14 g

SWEET POTATO SOUP

Serves 8 • Serving Size: 1 cup • Prep Time: 45 minutes

Cooking spray

4 medium sweet potatoes (about 6 oz each)

1 Tbsp olive oil

2 medium carrots, diced

2 medium celery stalks, diced

1 small onion, diced

1/2 tsp dried thyme

1/2 tsp ground black pepper

32 oz reduced-sodium, fat-free chicken broth

1/4 cup fat-free half-and-half, heated

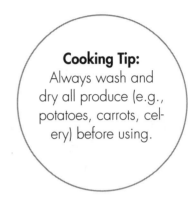

Cooking Tip:
Always wash and dry all produce (e.g., potatoes, carrots, celery) before using.

1. Preheat oven to 375°F.

2. Spray a baking sheet with cooking spray. Prick sweet potatoes on all sides with a fork and place them on the baking sheet. Spray sweet potatoes with cooking spray and bake for 45–50 minutes. Set aside to cool slightly.

3. Remove skin from sweet potatoes and cut into chunks. Discard skins.

4. Add oil to a large soup pot and heat over medium-high heat. Sauté carrots, celery, and onion for 3–4 minutes. Add remaining ingredients, except half-and-half. Bring to a simmer for 20 minutes.

5. Pour soup in a blender and puree until smooth (or puree soup with a handheld immersion blender directly in the pot). Pour soup 'back into soup pot and stir in half-and-half.

Exchanges/Choices
1 Starch

Calories 90
   Calories from Fat.....20
Total Fat ....2 g
   Saturated Fat ....0.3 g
   Trans Fat ....0 g
Cholesterol ....0 mg
Sodium ....295 mg
Total Carbohydrate ....16 g
   Dietary Fiber ....3 g
   Sugars ....7 g
Protein ....3 g

TERIYAKI TOFU

Serves 5 • Serving Size: 1/5th recipe • Prep Time: 15 minutes

14 oz extra-firm tofu, cut into chunks

1/4 cup reduced-sodium teriyaki sauce

1 Tbsp lite soy sauce

1 Tbsp sesame oil

4 oz whole-wheat vermicelli (spaghetti) noodles, uncooked

Cooking spray

3 cups broccoli florets

1 1/2 cups reduced-sodium, fat-free chicken broth

1 Tbsp cornstarch

Cooking Tip:
Be sure to buy extra-firm tofu, which is normally found in the produce section of the grocery store. It keeps its shape for stir-frying.

1. Add tofu to a medium bowl. Add teriyaki sauce, soy sauce, and sesame oil. Marinate in the refrigerator for 10 minutes.

2. Cook pasta according to package directions, omitting salt. Drain.

3. Add cooking spray to a wok or large sauté pan over high heat. Remove tofu from marinade, reserving marinade. Stir-fry tofu for 5–7 minutes or until it begins to brown.

4. Add broccoli and stir-fry another 4 minutes. Add reserved marinade and continue to stir-fry.

5. In a small bowl, whisk together chicken broth and cornstarch. Add to stir-fry and bring to a boil. Reduce to a simmer. Add cooked pasta to stir-fry and heat through.

Exchanges/Choices	
1 1/2 Starch	
1 Vegetable	
1 Lean Meat	
Calories	185
Calories from Fat	45
Total Fat	5 g
Saturated Fat	0.7 g
Trans Fat	0 g
Cholesterol	0 mg
Sodium	575 mg
Total Carbohydrate	24 g
Dietary Fiber	3 g
Sugars	5 g
Protein	11 g

the healthy carb diabetes cookbook

THAI CHICKEN PIZZA MEAL

Serves 8 • Serving Size: 1 slice • Prep Time: 25 minutes

Pizza

1 lb boneless, skinless chicken breast

1/2 tsp salt (*optional*)

1/4 tsp ground black pepper

Cooking spray

2 Tbsp creamy peanut butter

1/4 cup rice wine vinegar

3 Tbsp lite soy sauce

1 clove garlic, minced

1 (12-inch) prepackaged whole-wheat Italian pizza crust

1/2 cup reduced-fat, shredded mozzarella cheese

Salad

16 cups salad greens mix

16 tomato slices

1 cup diced cucumbers

8 Tbsp fat-free Italian salad dressing

Cooking Tip:
To add a little kick to this recipe, add 1/4 tsp crushed red pepper flakes to the peanut butter mixture.

1. Preheat oven to 375°F.

Exchanges/Choices
1 Starch
2 Vegetable
2 Lean Meat
1/2 Fat

Calories	235
Calories from Fat	65
Total Fat	7 g
Saturated Fat	2.4 g
Trans Fat	0 g
Cholesterol	35 mg
Sodium	675 mg
Total Carbohydrate	25 g
Dietary Fiber	4 g
Sugars	7 g
Protein	22 g

2. Season chicken with salt and pepper on both sides. Spray a baking sheet with cooking spray. Bake chicken for 25 minutes or until juices run clear. When cooled, chop chicken.

3. In a small saucepan, combine peanut butter, vinegar, soy sauce, and garlic. Bring to a simmer until melted and incorporated.

4. Spoon sauce evenly over premade crust. Top with chicken and mozzarella cheese.

5. Bake on rack in the oven for 20–25 minutes or until cheese is melted and bubbly.

6. While the pizza bakes, prepare the eight side salads (2 cups salad greens, 2 tomato slices, 2 Tbsp diced cucumbers, and 1 Tbsp salad dressing).

This recipe is high in sodium.

THREE-BEAN CHILI

Serves 9 • Serving Size: 1 cup • Prep Time: 20 minutes

Cooking spray

1 1/4 lb lean ground turkey breast

1 medium green bell pepper, diced

1 15-oz can light red kidney beans, drained and rinsed

1 15-oz can great northern beans, drained and rinsed

1 15-oz can black beans, drained and rinsed

2 14.5-oz cans no-salt-added diced tomatoes

1 15-oz can reduced-sodium tomato sauce

1 Tbsp chili powder

1/4 tsp cayenne pepper

1 tsp garlic powder

1 tsp onion powder

1/4 tsp ground black pepper

1. Add cooking spray to a large soup pot; cook turkey over medium-high heat, until it begins to brown. Drain fat.

2. Add green pepper to pot and sauté for 3–4 minutes. Add remaining ingredients and bring to a boil. Cover and simmer 10 minutes.

Nutrition Tip:
This one-pot meal is packed with good nutrition. It provides good sources of fiber, iron, vitamin C, and lycopene. Tomatoes provide lycopene, which is an antioxidant that may be helpful in reducing the risks of developing prostate cancer and heart disease.

Exchanges/Choices
1 Starch
2 Vegetable
2 Lean Meat
1 Fat

Calories 260
  Calories from Fat 65
Total Fat .... 7 g
  Saturated Fat .... 1.6 g
  Trans Fat .... 0 g
Cholesterol .... 45 mg
Sodium .... 245 mg
Total Carbohydrate .... 29 g
  Dietary Fiber .... 9 g
  Sugars .... 8 g
Protein .... 21 g

THANKSGIVING MEATLOAF

Serves 8 • Serving Size: 1 slice • Prep Time: 10 minutes

Cooking spray

1 cup corn bread or whole-wheat stuffing, cooked

1 lb ground turkey

1 egg

1/2 cup oats

1/2 tsp onion salt

3 Tbsp barbeque sauce (reserve 2 Tbsp)

1/2 Tbsp garlic powder

1/2 tsp ground black pepper

1/4 cup whole-berry cranberry sauce

1. Preheat oven to 375°F. Coat a 5 × 9-inch loaf pan with cooking spray.

2. Prepare stuffing according to package directions, omitting salt and butter. Set aside to cool.

3. In a large bowl, combine ground turkey, egg, oats, onion salt, 1 Tbsp barbeque sauce, garlic powder, and ground black pepper. Mix until all ingredients are incorporated; do not overmix.

4. In a small bowl, whisk together cranberry sauce and 2 Tbsp barbeque sauce.

5. Spread half of the turkey mixture evenly in the bottom of the pan. Using the back of a spoon, make a ditch through the center of the mixture without touching the bottom of the pan.

6. Spread stuffing evenly over the ditch; do not spread all the way to the sides of the pan.

Cooking Tip:
Serve this meatloaf with a vegetable like steamed green beans and you have an easy Thanksgiving-style meal any time of year!

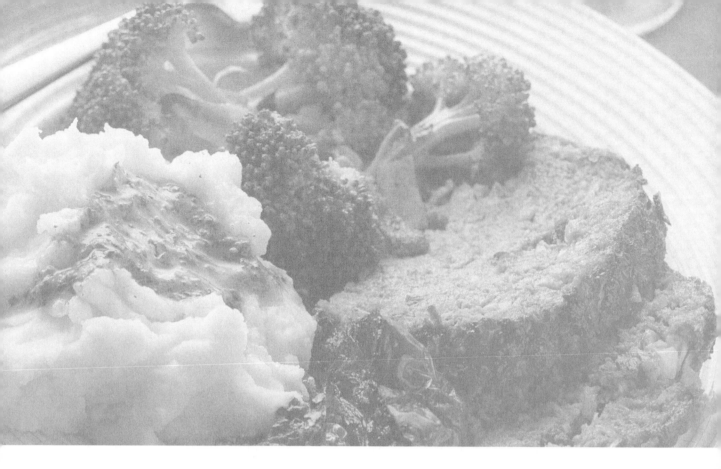

7. Add remaining turkey mixture over the stuffing and cover completely.

8. Bake meatloaf in oven for 30 minutes. Carefully remove the pan from the oven and spread the cranberry and barbeque sauce mixture over the top of the meatloaf. Return the pan to the oven for an additional 20 minutes. Remove from oven.

9. Let the meatloaf rest for 10–15 minutes before slicing.

Exchanges/Choices
1 Carbohydrate
2 Lean Meat

Calories 150
   Calories from Fat.....25
Total Fat .... 3 g
   Saturated Fat .... 0.8 g
   Trans Fat .... 0 g
Cholesterol .... 65 mg
Sodium .... 265 mg
Total Carbohydrate .... 16 g
   Dietary Fiber .... 1 g
   Sugars .... 7 g
Protein .... 15 g

the healthy carb diabetes cookbook

TILAPIA TACOS

Serves 8 • Serving Size: 1 taco • Prep Time: 20 minutes

3 limes, juiced

1 tsp hot sauce

1 Tbsp cilantro, chopped

4 tilapia fillets (about 1.35 lb)

1 tsp chili pepper

1/4 tsp salt (*optional*)

1/4 tsp ground black pepper

Cooking spray

8 small 6-inch whole-wheat tortillas,
  warmed

Sauce

1/2 cup fat-free sour cream

3 Tbsp canned diced green chilies

1. In a medium bowl, combine lime juice, hot sauce, and cilantro. Add fish to marinade and marinate in refrigerator for 15 minutes.

2. Remove fish from marinade and season with chili pepper, salt (optional), and pepper.

3. Coat a large sauté pan with cooking spray. Sauté fish over medium heat for 2–3 minutes on each side.

4. Remove fish from pan and shred into large pieces.

5. In a small bowl, combine sauce ingredients.

6. Evenly divide fish among eight tortillas. Top each taco with a dollop of sour cream sauce.

Exchanges/Choices
1 Starch
2 Lean Meat

Calories 175
  Calories from Fat 30
Total Fat .... 3.5 g
  Saturated Fat .... 0.8 g
  Trans Fat .... 0 g
Cholesterol .... 55 mg
Sodium .... 255 mg
Total Carbohydrate .... 16 g
  Dietary Fiber .... 2 g
  Sugars .... 2 g
Protein .... 18 g

Cooking Tip:
The fish in fish tacos is normally deep fried. This is a healthy and flavorful alternative to the fattening original.

PENNE WITH PEAR
AND GORGONZOLA ALFREDO

Serves 5 • Serving Size: 1 cup • Prep Time: 5 minutes

8 oz whole-wheat penne pasta, uncooked

2 tsp olive oil

2 medium pears, peeled, cored and diced

2 cloves garlic, minced

1/4 cup dry white wine

1 pint fat-free half-and-half

1/3 cup gorgonzola cheese, crumbled

1/2 tsp salt (*optional*)

1/8 tsp ground black pepper

Cooking Tip:
If you can't find gorgonzola cheese, substitute regular bleu cheese.

1. Cook pasta according to package directions, omitting salt. Drain.

2. In a medium sauté pan, heat oil over medium-high heat. Add pears and sauté 7 minutes or until they begin to soften.

3. Add garlic and sauté another minute. Add white wine and cook until wine is almost completely reduced.

4. Heat fat-free half-and-half in the microwave for 1 1/2 minutes. Pour over pears and bring to a low simmer. Do not boil. Simmer for 5–6 minutes. Using the back of a large spoon or plastic spatula, mash pears roughly in the sauce.

5. Stir in cheese, salt (optional), and pepper and simmer 1 more minute or until cheese is melted. Toss with cooked pasta.

Exchanges/Choices	
2 Starch	
1 Fruit	
1/2 Fat-Free Milk	
1 Fat	

Calories	300
Calories from Fat	55
Total Fat	6 g
Saturated Fat	2.5 g
Trans Fat	0 g
Cholesterol	10 mg
Sodium	205 mg
Total Carbohydrate	54 g
Dietary Fiber	7 g
Sugars	13 g
Protein	10 g

TUNA NOODLE CASSEROLE

Serves 10 • Serving Size: 1/10th recipe • Prep Time: 15 minutes

Cooking spray

2 cups whole-wheat penne pasta, uncooked

1 7-oz pkg chunk light tuna in water

1/8 tsp ground black pepper

24 oz frozen mixed vegetables in low-fat cheese sauce

1 10.75-oz can reduced-sodium cream of mushroom soup

1 cup nonfat milk

1/2 cup reduced-fat, shredded cheddar cheese

1. Preheat oven to 375°F. Coat a 9 × 13-inch baking dish with cooking spray.

2. Cook pasta according to package directions, omitting salt. Drain pasta and add to a large mixing bowl.

3. Add tuna, ground black pepper, frozen vegetables, cream of mushroom soup, and nonfat milk to pasta. Mix to incorporate.

4. Pour mixture into prepared baking dish. Sprinkle cheese evenly over the casserole and bake for 40 minutes or until bubbly and cheese is melted and beginning to brown.

Exchanges/Choices
1 Starch
1 Vegetable
1 Lean Meat

Calories	155
Calories from Fat	30
Total Fat	3.5 g
Saturated Fat	1.7 g
Trans Fat	0 g
Cholesterol	15 mg
Sodium	505 mg
Total Carbohydrate	22 g
Dietary Fiber	3 g
Sugars	4 g
Protein	11 g

Nutrition Tip:
Adding vegetables and whole-wheat pasta to this old favorite packs it full of fiber.

TURKEY CASSEROLE

Serves 7 • Serving Size: 1 cup • Prep Time: 20 minutes

Cooking spray

1 Tbsp canola oil

1 medium onion, peeled and diced

3 cups cooked turkey breast, diced

2 14.5-oz cans green beans, drained and rinsed

1 10.75-oz can reduced-fat cream of mushroom soup

1/2 cup fat-free sour cream

2/3 cup brown basmati/wild rice, cooked according to package directions

3/4 cup reduced-fat, shredded cheddar cheese

1. Preheat oven to 350°F. Coat a 3-quart casserole dish with cooking spray.

2. Heat oil in a small skillet over medium heat. Add onion and sauté until translucent, about 5 minutes. Remove from heat and transfer to a large bowl.

3. Add all remaining ingredients to bowl and mix together until thoroughly combined.

4. Pour mixture into casserole dish. Bake for 20–25 minutes or until bubbly. Let stand for a few minutes before serving.

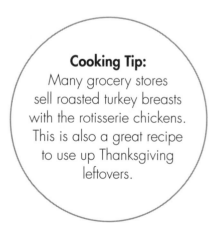

Cooking Tip:
Many grocery stores sell roasted turkey breasts with the rotisserie chickens. This is also a great recipe to use up Thanksgiving leftovers.

Exchanges/Choices
1 Starch
1 Vegetable
3 Lean Meat

Calories	250
Calories from Fat	65
Total Fat	7 g
Saturated Fat	2.4 g
Trans Fat	0 g
Cholesterol	60 mg
Sodium	490 mg
Total Carbohydrate	23 g
Dietary Fiber	3 g
Sugars	4 g
Protein	25 g

UNSTUFFED PEPPER SKILLET

Serves 8 • Serving Size: 1/8th recipe • Prep Time: 10 minutes

1 1/4 lb lean ground round

3 large green bell peppers, cut into 1-inch chunks

1 14.5-oz can no-salt-added diced tomatoes

1 15-oz can no-salt-added tomato sauce

1 1/2 cups water

1 tsp garlic powder

1/2 tsp onion salt

1/4 tsp ground black pepper

3/4 cup instant brown rice

1. Add ground round to a large deep skillet over medium-high heat and sauté until it begins to brown. Drain off any fat.

2. Add bell peppers and sauté for 5 minutes.

3. Add remaining ingredients and simmer covered for 35 minutes.

Exchanges/Choices
1 Starch
2 Vegetable
1 Lean Meat
1 Fat

Calories	215
Calories from Fat	55
Total Fat	6 g
Saturated Fat	2.3 g
Trans Fat	0.4 g
Cholesterol	45 mg
Sodium	170 mg
Total Carbohydrate	23 g
Dietary Fiber	3 g
Sugars	7 g
Protein	16 g

Cooking Tip:
This one-pot version is a great way to enjoy a traditionally time-consuming dish.

sides and appetizers

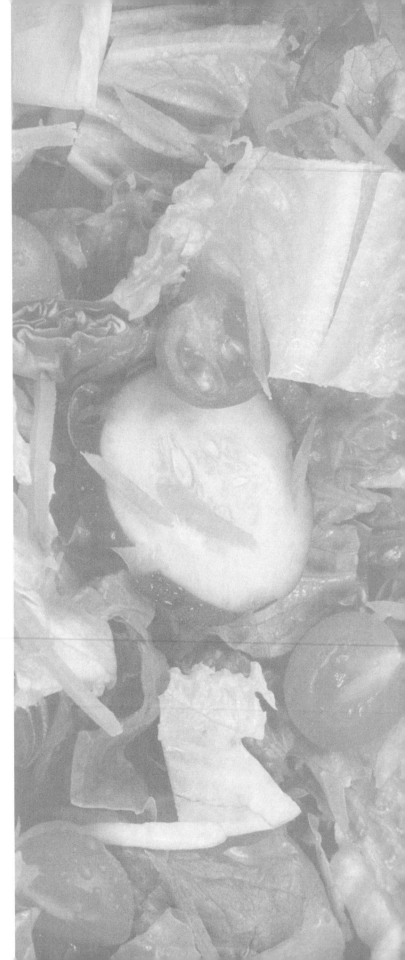

APRICOT PINE NUT COUSCOUS

Serves 10 • Serving Size: 1/2 cup • Prep Time: 10 minutes

2 cups reduced-sodium, fat-free chicken broth

1 1/2 cups whole-wheat couscous, uncooked

1/2 tsp salt (*optional*)

1/4 tsp ground black pepper

6 dried apricots, chopped

3 Tbsp low-sugar apricot preserves

1 green onion, thinly sliced

2 Tbsp pine nuts, toasted

1. In a medium saucepan, bring chicken broth to a boil. Add couscous. Cover and remove from heat. Let stand for 5 minutes and fluff with fork.

2. Add the remaining ingredients. Toss gently to coat.

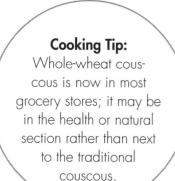

Cooking Tip:
Whole-wheat couscous is now in most grocery stores; it may be in the health or natural section rather than next to the traditional couscous.

Exchanges/Choices
1 Starch
1/2 Fruit

Calories	115
Calories from Fat	20
Total Fat	2 g
Saturated Fat	0.2 g
Trans Fat	0 g
Cholesterol	0 mg
Sodium	105 mg
Total Carbohydrate	22 g
Dietary Fiber	2 g
Sugars	4 g
Protein	4 g

BLACK BEAN DIP

Serves 15 • Serving Size: 1/15th recipe • Prep Time: 5 minutes

1 Tbsp olive oil

2 15-oz cans black beans, rinsed and drained

1 cup salsa

1 cup frozen corn

1 10-oz bag whole-wheat tortilla chips

1. Combine olive oil, black beans, salsa, and corn in a medium saucepan over medium-high heat. Simmer for 10 minutes.

2. Mash bean mixture and serve warm with whole-wheat tortilla chips.

Cooking Tip:
Make this dish as spicy as you like by purchasing mild, medium, or hot salsa.

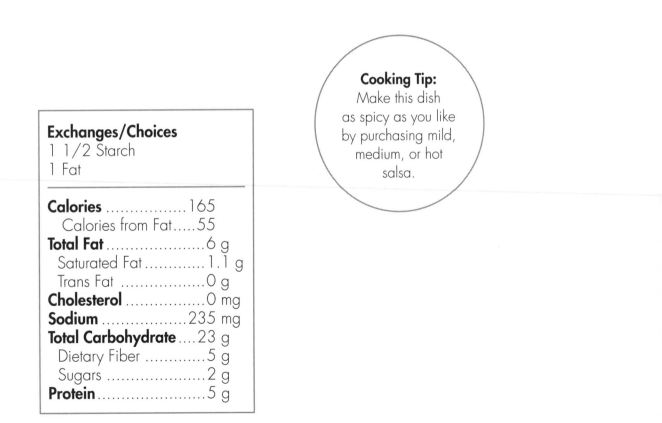

Exchanges/Choices
1 1/2 Starch
1 Fat

Calories 165
  Calories from Fat 55
Total Fat .... 6 g
  Saturated Fat .... 1.1 g
  Trans Fat .... 0 g
Cholesterol .... 0 mg
Sodium .... 235 mg
Total Carbohydrate .... 23 g
  Dietary Fiber .... 5 g
  Sugars .... 2 g
Protein .... 5 g

BLACK-EYED PEA SALAD

Serves 6 • Serving Size: 1/6th recipe • Prep Time: 10 minutes

2 Tbsp olive oil

4 Tbsp red wine vinegar

2 15-oz cans black-eyed peas, drained and rinsed

1/2 red bell pepper, diced

2 green onions, chopped

1 jalapeño pepper, seeded and diced

2 Tbsp fresh parsley, chopped

1/4 tsp garlic salt

1/4 tsp ground black pepper

1. In a small bowl, whisk together olive oil and vinegar.

2. In a large bowl, mix together the remaining ingredients. Pour dressing over salad and toss well to coat.

Cooking Tip:
If you prefer things less spicy, use one whole red pepper and omit the jalapeño pepper. This salad can be made the day before and refrigerated until serving.

Exchanges/Choices
1 1/2 Starch
1 Fat

Calories 160
  Calories from Fat..... 45
Total Fat .... 5 g
  Saturated Fat .... 0.6 g
  Trans Fat .... 0 g
Cholesterol .... 0 mg
Sodium .... 210 mg
Total Carbohydrate .... 23 g
  Dietary Fiber .... 7 g
  Sugars .... 5 g
Protein .... 8 g

BREADED ZUCCHINI

Serves 7 • Serving Size: 1/2 cup • Prep Time: 10 minutes

Cooking spray

2 egg whites

1/2 cup cornmeal

1/4 cup grated Parmesan cheese

1/2 tsp garlic powder

1/4 tsp ground black pepper

3 medium zucchini, cut into 2-inch pieces

1. Preheat oven to 375°F. Coat a baking sheet with cooking spray.

2. In a small bowl, whisk together the egg whites. In a separate bowl, add cornmeal, Parmesan cheese, garlic powder, and ground black pepper; stir to incorporate.

3. Dip each zucchini piece in egg mixture and then in cornmeal to coat.

4. Evenly distribute the coated zucchini over the baking sheet and spray zucchini with cooking spray.

5. Bake for 20–25 minutes or until golden brown.

Exchanges/Choices
1/2 Starch
1 Vegetable

Calories	70
Calories from Fat	15
Total Fat	1.5 g
Saturated Fat	0.6 g
Trans Fat	0 g
Cholesterol	5 mg
Sodium	50 mg
Total Carbohydrate	11 g
Dietary Fiber	2 g
Sugars	2 g
Protein	4 g

Nutrition Tip:
Cornmeal is an underutilized whole-grain source. Most people are unsure of how to cook with it, and this zucchini recipe is just one example of its great use.

BROCCOLI AND CAULIFLOWER CASSEROLE

Serves 8 • Serving Size: 1/8th recipe • Prep Time: 25 minutes

Cooking spray

Water (about 1 cup)

2 cups broccoli florets

1 head cauliflower, chopped

1 egg

1/2 cup fat-free half-and-half

1/2 cup + 2 Tbsp reduced-fat, shredded
  cheddar cheese

1/2 tsp salt (*optional*)

1/4 tsp ground black pepper

Nutrition Tip:
Broccoli and cauliflower are both part of the cruciferous vegetable family, which may protect against certain types of cancer.

1. Preheat oven to 375°F. Coat a 9 × 13-inch baking dish with cooking spray.

2. In a large, deep sauté pan, add water. Add broccoli and cauliflower. Bring to a boil. Reduce to simmer. Cover tightly with lid and steam for 20 minutes or until soft.

3. Drain water from broccoli and cauliflower, making sure all water is gone.

4. In a large bowl, mash together the broccoli and cauliflower. Stir in egg, fat-free half-and-half, 1/2 cup cheese, salt (optional), and pepper.

5. Pour cauliflower and broccoli mixture in prepared dish and spread evenly. Sprinkle remaining 2 Tbsp cheese over the top and bake for 20 minutes or until cheese is melted and beginning to brown.

Exchanges/Choices
1 Vegetable
1/2 Fat

Calories 65
  Calories from Fat..... 25
Total Fat .... 3 g
  Saturated Fat .... 1.4 g
  Trans Fat .... 0 g
Cholesterol .... 35 mg
Sodium .... 125 mg
Total Carbohydrate ...... 6 g
  Dietary Fiber .... 2 g
  Sugars .... 3 g
Protein .... 5 g

the healthy carb diabetes cookbook

BROWN RICE PILAF

Serves 10 • Serving Size: 1/2 cup • Prep Time: 20 minutes

2 tsp canola oil

Cooking spray

2 small carrots, finely diced

2 stalks celery, finely diced

1 cup mushrooms, chopped

1/4 cup slivered almonds

2 cups instant brown rice

1 14.5-oz can reduced-sodium, fat-free chicken broth

1/2 tsp salt (*optional*)

1/4 tsp ground black pepper

1. Add canola oil and a generous amount of cooking spray to a medium saucepan.

2. Sauté carrots, celery, mushrooms, and almonds for 3–4 minutes or until they begin to soften. Add remaining ingredients and bring to a boil.

3. Reduce to a simmer, cover, and cook for an additional 15–20 minutes or until rice is tender. Fluff with a fork.

Exchanges/Choices
2 Starch
1/2 Fat

Calories	170
Calories from Fat	30
Total Fat	3.5 g
Saturated Fat	0.2 g
Trans Fat	0 g
Cholesterol	0 mg
Sodium	130 mg
Total Carbohydrate	32 g
Dietary Fiber	2 g
Sugars	1 g
Protein	5 g

Cooking Tip:
This side dish is a great accompaniment to any meal.

BRUSCHETTA

Serves 9 • Serving Size: 2 pieces • Prep Time: 10 minutes

Cooking spray

2 Tbsp olive oil, divided

2 tsp garlic, minced

4 Tbsp balsamic vinegar

1/4 tsp salt (optional)

1/8 tsp ground black pepper

2 cups tomatoes, seeded and chopped

1/2 cup onion, finely chopped

1/4 cup fresh basil, chopped

1 whole-wheat baguette

Nutrition Tip:
A whole-wheat baguette can be found in your grocer's bakery section. Although it may be difficult to find a 100% whole-wheat baguette, a wheat baguette will still offer more fiber than the traditional white baguette.

1. Preheat oven to 375°F. Coat a baking sheet with cooking spray.

2. Add 1 Tbsp olive oil to a small sauté pan over medium heat. Add garlic and sauté for 1 minute.

3. In a small bowl, combine olive oil and garlic mixture with balsamic vinegar, salt (optional), pepper, tomatoes, onion, and basil.

4. Let mixture marinate in refrigerator for 30 minutes.

5. Slice whole-wheat baguette into 18 pieces. Lightly brush remaining olive oil on each piece.

6. Line baguette pieces on baking sheet and bake for 10–12 minutes or until toasted.

7. Top each baguette piece with equal amounts of tomato mixture.

Exchanges/Choices
2 Starch
1/2 Fat

Calories	180
Calories from Fat	40
Total Fat	4.5 g
Saturated Fat	0.8 g
Trans Fat	0 g
Cholesterol	0 mg
Sodium	250 mg
Total Carbohydrate	30 g
Dietary Fiber	3 g
Sugars	4 g
Protein	5 g

the healthy carb diabetes cookbook

BRUSSELS SPROUTS WITH BACON

Serves 6 • Serving Size: 1/2 cup • Prep Time: 2 minutes

5 slices turkey bacon, cut into 1/2-inch pieces

1 Tbsp trans-fat-free margarine

2 10-oz pkg frozen Brussels sprouts, thawed

1. In a skillet, cook bacon over medium-high heat until slightly crisp.

2. Add margarine to skillet and melt. Add Brussels sprouts and sauté for 5–7 minutes.

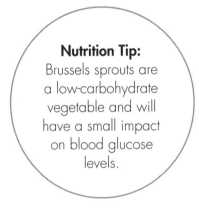

Nutrition Tip:
Brussels sprouts are a low-carbohydrate vegetable and will have a small impact on blood glucose levels.

Exchanges/Choices
2 Vegetable
1 Fat

Calories	80
Calories from Fat	40
Total Fat	4.5 g
Saturated Fat	1.1 g
Trans Fat	0 g
Cholesterol	10 mg
Sodium	175 mg
Total Carbohydrate	8 g
Dietary Fiber	4 g
Sugars	2 g
Protein	5 g

CALIFORNIA CORN SALAD

Serves 5 • Serving Size: 1/5th recipe • Prep Time: 10 minutes

2 limes, juiced

1 orange, juiced

1 Tbsp chopped cilantro

1 Tbsp Splenda

2 Tbsp olive oil

1 5-oz bag field green salad mix

1 cup fresh or frozen corn kernels (if frozen, thawed)

1 avocado, peeled, seeded, and sliced

1. In a small bowl, whisk together lime juice, orange juice, cilantro, Splenda, and olive oil. Set aside.

2. In a medium bowl, toss together field greens, corn kernels, and avocado.

3. Pour dressing over salad mixture and toss well to coat evenly.

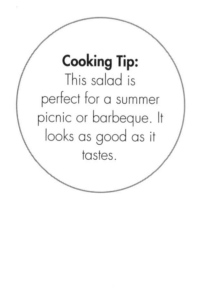

Cooking Tip:
This salad is perfect for a summer picnic or barbeque. It looks as good as it tastes.

Exchanges/Choices
1/2 Starch
1 Vegetable
2 Fat

Calories	140
Calories from Fat.....	90
Total Fat..................	10 g
Saturated Fat............	1.4 g
Trans Fat	0 g
Cholesterol	0 mg
Sodium	10 mg
Total Carbohydrate....	13 g
Dietary Fiber	3 g
Sugars	4 g
Protein......................	2 g

CHEESY CAULIFLOWER MASH

Serves 8 • Serving Size: 1/2 cup • Prep Time: 20 minutes

1 large head cauliflower

1/4 cup fat-free half-and-half, heated

3/4 cup reduced-fat, shredded cheddar cheese

1/4 tsp salt (*optional*)

1/4 tsp ground black pepper

1. Over high heat, add water to a large soup pot until it goes up the side about 1 inch. Add cauliflower and cover. Steam cauliflower until very soft. Drain water.

2. Add all remaining ingredients to cauliflower pot. Use an electric mixer or immersion blender on low speed to beat together all ingredients until smooth.

Cooking Tip:
You can add turkey bacon to this recipe for a taste similar to bacon cheese mashed potatoes.

Exchanges/Choices
1 Vegetable
1/2 Fat

Calories 60
  Calories from Fat.....20
Total Fat ....2.5 g
  Saturated Fat.............1.4 g
  Trans Fat ....0 g
Cholesterol ....10 mg
Sodium ....125 mg
Total Carbohydrate......6 g
  Dietary Fiber ....3 g
  Sugars ....3 g
Protein......................5 g

CITRUS SALAD

Serves 5 • Serving Size: 1/5th recipe • Prep Time: 10 minutes

5 oz mixed baby salad greens

1/2 cup orange segments

1/2 cup ruby red grapefruit segments

2 Tbsp rice wine vinegar

2 Tbsp olive oil

1/4 cup orange juice

1/4 cup ruby red grapefruit juice

1/4 tsp salt (*optional*)

8 Tbsp almond slivers, toasted

1. In a medium bowl, toss together salad greens, orange segments, and grapefruit segments.

2. In a small bowl, whisk together rice wine vinegar, olive oil, orange juice, grapefruit juice, and salt (optional).

3. Pour dressing over salad and toss again to coat evenly. Sprinkle with toasted almond slivers.

Nutrition Tip:
Nuts and almonds can be a tasty and healthy addition to a salad. Nuts are a good source of healthy unsaturated fats, but should be eaten in moderation to control calorie intake. You only need a small amount of nuts for added flavor and crunch.

Exchanges/Choices
1/2 Fruit
2 1/2 Fat

Calories 155
  Calories from Fat... 110
Total Fat .... 12 g
  Saturated Fat .... 1.3 g
  Trans Fat .... 0 g
Cholesterol .... 0 mg
Sodium .... 5 mg
Total Carbohydrate .... 10 g
  Dietary Fiber .... 3 g
  Sugars .... 7 g
Protein .... 4 g

COCKTAIL MEATBALLS

Serves 8 • Serving Size: 3 meatballs • Prep Time: 25 minutes

Meatballs

1 lb lean ground turkey breast

1 1/2 tsp dried minced onion

1 egg, slightly beaten

1/2 tsp garlic salt

1/4 tsp ground black pepper

1/3 cup old-fashioned rolled oats

Sauce

1/2 cup low-sugar grape jelly

1 8-oz can no-salt-added tomato sauce

1/2 cup chili sauce

2 tsp hot sauce (*optional*)

1. Preheat oven to 375°F.

2. In a medium bowl, mix meatball ingredients together. Shape into 1-inch balls.

3. Place meatballs on baking sheet and bake for 25 minutes, until brown and done.

4. In a large saucepan, combine sauce ingredients. Bring to a boil over medium heat. Reduce heat and simmer 5 minutes, stirring occasionally.

5. Add meatballs to sauce and stir to coat. Simmer over medium heat for 10 minutes, stirring occasionally. Serve warm.

Exchanges/Choices
1 Carbohydrate
2 Lean Meat

Calories	135
Calories from Fat	10
Total Fat	1 g
Saturated Fat	0.3 g
Trans Fat	0 g
Cholesterol	65 mg
Sodium	320 mg
Total Carbohydrate	14 g
Dietary Fiber	1 g
Sugars	8 g
Protein	15 g

Nutrition Tip:
This classic appetizer is made healthy with oats, turkey, and low-sugar jelly for reduced fat and carbohydrate content.

CRABBIES

Serves 20 • Serving Size: 2 pieces • Prep Time: 5 minutes

Cooking spray

1 8-oz can lump crab meat

8 oz light cream cheese with chives and onions

5 whole-wheat English muffins

1. Preheat oven to 375°F. Coat a baking sheet with cooking spray.

2. In a small bowl, combine crab and cream cheese. Mix well. Divide mixture among 10 English muffin halves.

3. Place English muffin halves with crab side up on baking sheets.

4. Bake for 30 minutes.

5. Remove from oven and cut each half into fourths. Serve warm.

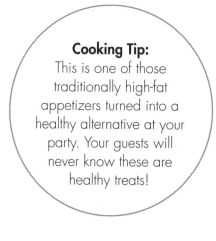

Cooking Tip:
This is one of those traditionally high-fat appetizers turned into a healthy alternative at your party. Your guests will never know these are healthy treats!

Exchanges/Choices
1/2 Starch
1/2 Fat

Calories 65
  Calories from Fat.....20
Total Fat ....2 g
  Saturated Fat ....1.2 g
  Trans Fat ....0 g
Cholesterol ....15 mg
Sodium ....180 mg
Total Carbohydrate ......7 g
  Dietary Fiber ....1 g
  Sugars ....2 g
Protein ....5 g

CRANBERRY WALNUT SALAD

Serves 5 • Serving Size: 1/5th recipe • Prep Time: 10 minutes

5 oz field green salad mix

1/4 cup dried cranberries

1/4 cup walnuts, chopped and toasted

1 cup shredded carrots

4 green onions, chopped

3 Tbsp balsamic vinegar

1 Tbsp olive oil

1 Tbsp Splenda

1/4 tsp salt (*optional*)

1/4 tsp ground black pepper

1. In a large bowl, toss together the field greens, cranberries, walnuts, carrots, and green onions.

2. In a small bowl, whisk together balsamic vinegar, olive oil, Splenda, salt (optional), and pepper.

3. Pour dressing over the salad and toss to coat evenly.

Exchanges/Choices
1/2 Fruit
1 Vegetable
1 1/2 Fat

Calories	110
Calories from Fat	65
Total Fat	7 g
Saturated Fat	0.7 g
Trans Fat	0 g
Cholesterol	0 mg
Sodium	25 mg
Total Carbohydrate	12 g
Dietary Fiber	2 g
Sugars	8 g
Protein	2 g

Cooking Tip:
This is a beautiful salad to serve at a holiday party.

CUCUMBER SHRIMP CANAPÉS

Serves 8 • Serving Size: 2 pieces • Prep Time: 5 minutes

1 lb cooked peeled shrimp, finely chopped

1/4 cup nonfat plain yogurt

1/4 cup light mayonnaise

1 Tbsp + 1 tsp dried dill, divided

1/4 tsp salt (*optional*)

Dash ground black pepper

1 large cucumber, cut into 16 1/4-inch-thick slices

1. In a medium bowl, combine all ingredients except cucumber and 1 tsp dill.

2. Spoon even amounts of shrimp mixture over each cucumber slice.

3. Sprinkle canapés with remaining 1 tsp of dill.

Cooking Tip:
Hothouse cucumbers, also know as seedless or European cucumbers, work great for this recipe. They are usually individually wrapped in plastic in the produce section of your grocery store.

Exchanges/Choices
2 Lean Meat

Calories	90
Calories from Fat	25
Total Fat	3 g
Saturated Fat	0.6 g
Trans Fat	0 g
Cholesterol	115 mg
Sodium	200 mg
Total Carbohydrate	3 g
Dietary Fiber	0 g
Sugars	1 g
Protein	13 g

CUCUMBER TOMATO SALAD WITH FETA

Serves 6 • Serving Size: 1/6th recipe • Prep Time: 25 minutes

5 plum (roma) tomatoes, seeded and cut into 1/2-inch chunks

2 large cucumbers, peeled, seeded, and cut into 1/2-inch chunks

3 oz reduced-fat feta cheese, crumbled

1/4 cup + 1 Tbsp rice wine vinegar

1 Tbsp olive oil

1/4 tsp crushed red pepper flakes

1 Tbsp dried dill

1 Tbsp Splenda

1. In a large bowl, combine tomatoes, cucumbers, and feta.

2. In a small bowl, whisk together remaining ingredients and pour over tomato salad.

3. Toss gently to coat.

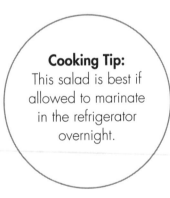

Cooking Tip:
This salad is best if allowed to marinate in the refrigerator overnight.

Exchanges/Choices	
1 Vegetable	
1 Fat	

Calories	75
Calories from Fat	40
Total Fat	4.5 g
Saturated Fat	1.6 g
Trans Fat	0 g
Cholesterol	5 mg
Sodium	200 mg
Total Carbohydrate	6 g
Dietary Fiber	2 g
Sugars	4 g
Protein	4 g

FIVE-MINUTE SPINACH DIP

Serves 16 • Serving Size: 2 Tbsp • Prep Time: 5 minutes

1 10-oz pkg chopped frozen spinach, thawed and drained

8 oz light sour cream

8 oz nonfat plain yogurt

1/2 pkg (0.7-oz pkg) vegetable soup mix

2 green onions, chopped

1/4 tsp garlic powder

1. In a medium bowl, combine all ingredients and mix well.

2. Chill in refrigerator for 2 hours before serving.

3. Serve with whole-wheat crackers or vegetables.

Cooking Tip:
This recipe is also great with toasted whole-wheat pitas.

Exchanges/Choices
1/2 Carbohydrate

Calories 35
　Calories from Fat 15
Total Fat .... 1.5 g
　Saturated Fat .... 1 g
　Trans Fat .... 0 g
Cholesterol .... 5 mg
Sodium .... 60 mg
Total Carbohydrate ...... 3 g
　Dietary Fiber .... 1 g
　Sugars .... 2 g
Protein .... 2 g

GREEN BEAN BUNDLES

Serves 11 • Serving Size: 1 bundle • Prep Time: 15 minutes

Cooking spray

1 lb fresh green beans

11 strips turkey bacon

1/4 tsp garlic salt

1/8 tsp ground black pepper

1 Tbsp trans-fat-free margarine

3 Tbsp Splenda Brown Sugar Blend

Cooking Tip:
These green bean bundles would be a perfect addition to Thanksgiving dinner.

1. Preheat oven to 375°F. Coat a large baking dish or baking sheet with cooking spray.

2. Blanch green beans in boiling water for 3 minutes. Drain and rinse in cold water.

3. Microwave turkey bacon strips for 2 1/2 minutes.

4. Take seven green beans and wrap one slice of turkey bacon around them, forming a bundle. Place green bean bundle in a baking dish.

5. Repeat procedure for remaining 10 bundles. Sprinkle green beans with garlic salt and pepper.

6. In a small bowl, mix together margarine and Brown Sugar Blend. Drop Brown Sugar Blend mixture evenly on top of each green bean bundle.

7. Bake at 375°F for 20 minutes.

Exchanges/Choices
1/2 Carbohydrate
1/2 Fat

Calories	70
Calories from Fat	35
Total Fat	4 g
Saturated Fat	1 g
Trans Fat	0 g
Cholesterol	15 mg
Sodium	210 mg
Total Carbohydrate	6 g
Dietary Fiber	1 g
Sugars	4 g
Protein	3 g

GREEN RICE

Serves 4 • Serving Size: 1/4th recipe • Prep Time: 5 minutes

2 tsp olive oil

3 tomatillos, diced small

1 cup cilantro leaves, finely chopped

1/4 tsp garlic salt

1 cup instant brown rice

1 cup reduced-sodium, fat-free chicken broth

1. Heat oil in a medium saucepan over medium-high heat.

2. Add tomatillos and sauté for 5 minutes or until soft. Add remaining ingredients and bring to a boil.

3. Reduce to a simmer and cook covered for 10 minutes or until rice is tender.

4. Stir well after cooking.

Cooking Tip:
Tomatillos are a fruit that are also called Mexican green tomatoes. They look like small green tomatoes except for a thin leafy husk. Be sure to remove this husk and wash the fruit before use.

Exchanges/Choices
2 1/2 Starch

Calories 200
  Calories from Fat.....35
Total Fat ....4 g
  Saturated Fat ....0.3 g
  Trans Fat ....0 g
Cholesterol ....0 mg
Sodium ....225 mg
Total Carbohydrate ....38 g
  Dietary Fiber ....2 g
  Sugars ....2 g
Protein ....5 g

GUACAMOLE

Serves 8 • Serving Size: 2 Tbsp • Prep Time: 5 minutes

2 medium avocados, pitted

2 plum (roma) tomatoes, seeded and chopped

1/2 small lime, juiced

1/2 tsp garlic powder

Pinch ground black pepper

1/4 tsp salt (*optional*)

1. In a medium bowl, combine all ingredients and mix well.

2. Serve with baked whole-wheat tortilla chips.

Nutrition Tip:
Avocados are a good source of monounsaturated fat, which is the good fat for a healthy heart. Just be sure to watch your portion size because they are high in calories.

Exchanges/Choices
1 Vegetable
1 Fat

Calories 65
  Calories from Fat.....55
Total Fat....................6 g
  Saturated Fat............0.8 g
  Trans Fat ....0 g
Cholesterol ....0 mg
Sodium ....0 mg
Total Carbohydrate......4 g
  Dietary Fiber ....3 g
  Sugars ....1 g
Protein.......................1 g

HOT 'N' SPICY CRAB DIP

Serves 16 • Serving Size: 2 Tbsp • Prep Time: 5 minutes

Cooking spray

4 6-oz cans lump crabmeat, drained

1 clove garlic, minced

1 4-oz can diced green chiles, drained

1 cup reduced-fat, shredded Monterey Jack cheese

1 tsp Worcestershire sauce

1 tsp hot sauce

1/3 cup light mayonnaise

2 Tbsp nonfat plain yogurt

2 Tbsp grated Parmesan cheese

1. Preheat oven to 350°F. Spray a 9-inch round baking dish with cooking spray.

2. In a medium bowl, combine all ingredients except Parmesan cheese. Mix gently.

3. Spread the crabmeat mixture into baking dish. Sprinkle Parmesan cheese on top of crabmeat mixture.

4. Bake for 25 minutes or until golden brown. Remove from oven and let sit 5 minutes before serving.

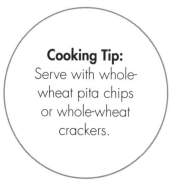

Cooking Tip:
Serve with whole-wheat pita chips or whole-wheat crackers.

Exchanges/Choices
1 Lean Meat
1/2 Fat

Calories	70
Calories from Fat	30
Total Fat	3.5 g
Saturated Fat	1.4 g
Trans Fat	0 g
Cholesterol	35 mg
Sodium	225 mg
Total Carbohydrate	1 g
Dietary Fiber	0 g
Sugars	0 g
Protein	8 g

MARINATED CAPRESE SALAD

Serves 8 • Serving Size: about 1/2 cup • Prep Time: 20 minutes

6 plum (roma) tomatoes, seeded and cut into 1/2-inch chunks

1 Tbsp olive oil

3 Tbsp balsamic vinegar

1 oz fresh basil (about 15 leaves), chopped

1/4 tsp salt (*optional*)

Dash ground black pepper

3 oz fresh mozzarella cheese, cut into small chunks

1. In a large bowl combine all ingredients. Mix well.

2. Let marinate for 1 hour in the refrigerator.

Cooking Tip:
Fresh mozzarella is found in the deli case or with the specialty cheeses. It is formed into balls and packed in water. Be sure to drain the water before use.

Exchanges/Choices
1 Vegetable
1/2 Fat

Calories	60
Calories from Fat	30
Total Fat	3.5 g
Saturated Fat	1.4 g
Trans Fat	0 g
Cholesterol	5 mg
Sodium	60 mg
Total Carbohydrate	4 g
Dietary Fiber	1 g
Sugars	3 g
Protein	3 g

MARINATED EGGPLANT

Serves 5 • Serving Size: 1/2 cup • Prep Time: 5 minutes

Cooking spray
1 medium eggplant, cut into 1-inch cubes
1 Tbsp lite soy sauce
2 Tbsp canola oil
1 Tbsp rice wine vinegar
2 Tbsp Splenda Brown Sugar Blend
1/2 tsp garlic powder

1. Preheat oven to 375°F. Coat a baking sheet with cooking spray.

2. In a medium bowl, combine all other ingredients. Let eggplant marinate in refrigerator for 30 minutes.

3. Spread eggplant evenly on baking sheet and roast in oven for 20 minutes.

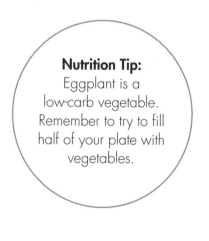

Nutrition Tip:
Eggplant is a low-carb vegetable. Remember to try to fill half of your plate with vegetables.

Exchanges/Choices		
2 Vegetable		
1/2 Fat		

Calories	65
Calories from Fat	25
Total Fat	3 g
Saturated Fat	0.2 g
Trans Fat	0 g
Cholesterol	0 mg
Sodium	60 mg
Total Carbohydrate	10 g
Dietary Fiber	2 g
Sugars	5 g
Protein	1 g

the healthy carb diabetes cookbook

MARINATED PEPPER SALAD

Serves 6 • Serving Size: 1/2 cup • Prep Time: 15 minutes

1 medium green bell pepper, cut into 1/2-inch strips

1 medium red bell pepper, cut into 1/2-inch strips

1 medium orange bell pepper, cut into 1/2-inch strips

1/2 tsp dried oregano

1/4 tsp crushed red pepper flakes

1 1/2 Tbsp Splenda

1 Tbsp olive oil

1/4 cup red wine vinegar

1/4 tsp salt (*optional*)

1/4 tsp ground black pepper

1. In a large bowl, combine all ingredients.

2. Let marinate for 1 hour in the refrigerator.

Exchanges/Choices
1 Vegetable
1/2 Fat

Calories	40
Calories from Fat.....	20
Total Fat	2.5 g
Saturated Fat	0.3 g
Trans Fat	0 g
Cholesterol	0 mg
Sodium	0 mg
Total Carbohydrate	5 g
Dietary Fiber	1 g
Sugars	3 g
Protein	1 g

Cooking Tip:
Try experimenting with different colors of peppers for this salad: red, yellow, orange, green, and even purple!

MEDITERRANEAN TORTELLINI SALAD

Serves 16 • Serving Size: 1/2 cup • Prep Time: 20 minutes

Salad

2 9-oz pkg refrigerated whole-wheat
tortellini

1 pint grape tomatoes, halved

3 oz fat-free feta cheese, crumbled

1/4 red onion, finely diced

Dressing

3 Tbsp olive oil

1/3 cup red wine vinegar

1 Tbsp Dijon mustard

1/4 tsp ground black pepper

1/2 tsp garlic powder

1/2 tsp Splenda

1. Cook tortellini according to package directions, omitting salt. Drain.

2. In a medium bowl, combine salad ingredients.

3. In a small bowl, whisk together dressing ingredients.

4. Pour dressing over tortellini salad and toss gently to coat.

Cooking Tip:
Cooked chopped chicken breast could be added to this salad to make it a meal.

Exchanges/Choices	
1 Starch	
1 Fat	

Calories	130
Calories from Fat	40
Total Fat	4.5 g
Saturated Fat	1.4 g
Trans Fat	0 g
Cholesterol	10 mg
Sodium	250 mg
Total Carbohydrate	17 g
Dietary Fiber	1 g
Sugars	2 g
Protein	6 g

PROSCIUTTO-WRAPPED ASPARAGUS

Serves 5 • Serving Size: 1 bundle • Prep Time: 10 minutes

1 1/2 lb asparagus spears, ends trimmed

2 tsp olive oil

1/8 tsp ground black pepper

1/8 tsp garlic powder

5 slices prosciutto

1. Preheat oven to 400°F.

2. In a large bowl or dish, toss asparagus with olive oil. Season the asparagus with pepper and garlic powder.

3. Bundle about 4–5 asparagus spears together. Use a slice of prosciutto to wrap the bundle and secure the spears with a toothpick. Repeat the process for the remaining four bundles.

4. Place asparagus bundles on baking sheet and bake for 12 minutes.

Exchanges/Choices
1 Vegetable
1 Lean Meat

Calories 70
  Calories from Fat.....30
Total Fat.....................3.5 g
  Saturated Fat.............0.7 g
  Trans Fat ....0 g
Cholesterol ....10 mg
Sodium ....260 mg
Total Carbohydrate......5 g
  Dietary Fiber ....2 g
  Sugars ....2 g
Protein........................7 g

Nutrition Tip:
Asparagus is a great source of folic acid, fiber, and potassium.

ROASTED BUTTERNUT SQUASH

Serves 6 • Serving Size: 1/2 cup • Prep Time: 5 minutes

1 large butternut squash (about 2 lb), halved and seeded

Cooking spray

3 Tbsp light cream cheese with chives and onions

1/4 tsp salt (*optional*)

1/4 tsp ground black pepper

1. Preheat oven to 400°F. Spray both sides of squash with cooking spray and place face down in glass baking dish. Bake for 1 hour.

2. Remove squash from oven. Scoop squash into a medium bowl and discard skin.

3. Add cream cheese, salt (optional), and pepper. Whip with a whisk until smooth.

Nutrition Tip:
Using the light cream cheese instead of butter or cream is an easy way to cut out a lot of fat without sacrificing flavor. It works great with mashed potatoes as well.

Exchanges/Choices
1 Starch

Calories	60
Calories from Fat	10
Total Fat	1 g
Saturated Fat	0.7 g
Trans Fat	0 g
Cholesterol	5 mg
Sodium	45 mg
Total Carbohydrate	12 g
Dietary Fiber	1 g
Sugars	3 g
Protein	2 g

ROASTED EGGPLANT DIP

Serves 9 • Serving Size: 2 Tbsp • Prep Time: 5 minutes

2 Tbsp olive oil, divided

1 large eggplant (about 1 1/4 lb), peeled and cut into 1-inch cubes

1/2 tsp garlic salt

1/4 tsp ground black pepper

1/4 tsp salt (*optional*)

3 Tbsp grated Parmesan cheese

1. Preheat oven to 375°F.

2. In a medium bowl, toss 1 Tbsp olive oil and eggplant cubes together to coat evenly.

3. Spread evenly on a baking sheet. Bake for 20–25 minutes or until eggplant begins to brown.

4. Add roasted eggplant and remaining ingredients, including remaining tablespoon of olive oil, to a blender or food processor and puree until smooth. Serve warm.

Exchanges/Choices
1 Vegetable
1/2 Fat

Calories	50
Calories from Fat	30
Total Fat	3.5 g
Saturated Fat	0.8 g
Trans Fat	0 g
Cholesterol	0 mg
Sodium	85 mg
Total Carbohydrate	4 g
Dietary Fiber	1 g
Sugars	2 g
Protein	1 g

Cooking Tip:
Serve this great party dip with whole-wheat pita chips or whole-grain tortilla chip. Both are sure to be a hit!

ROASTED VEGETABLES

Serves 8 • Serving Size: 1/2 cup • Prep Time: 10 minutes

Cooking spray
1 lb asparagus, cut into 1-inch pieces
2 zucchini, diced
1 medium eggplant (about 1 lb), diced
1 1/2 Tbsp olive oil
1 tsp garlic powder
1/4 tsp ground black pepper

1. Preheat oven to 375°F. Coat a large baking dish with cooking spray.

2. In large bowl, mix together all ingredients. Spread mixture evenly in baking dish.

3. Bake 40–45 minutes or until brown and roasted.

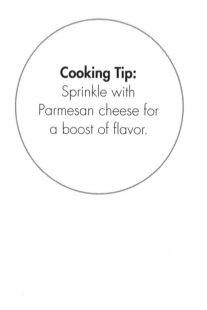

Cooking Tip:
Sprinkle with
Parmesan cheese for
a boost of flavor.

Exchanges/Choices	
2 Vegetable	
1/2 Fat	

Calories	60
Calories from Fat	25
Total Fat	3 g
Saturated Fat	0.4 g
Trans Fat	0 g
Cholesterol	0 mg
Sodium	5 mg
Total Carbohydrate	8 g
Dietary Fiber	3 g
Sugars	3 g
Protein	2 g

SAUTÉED PEAS

Serves 4 • Serving Size: 1/3 cup • Prep Time: 2 minutes

2 tsp olive oil

1 garlic clove, minced

1 9-oz box frozen peas, thawed

1/4 tsp ground black pepper

1. Heat oil in medium sauté pan over medium heat.

2. Add garlic and sauté 30 seconds.

3. Add peas and pepper and sauté until heated through, about 3 to 5 minutes.

Nutrition Tip:
Peas provide about 15 grams of carbohydrate (1 Carb Choice) per 1/2 cup, but that does not mean you should avoid them. Count them toward your allotted carbohydrate intake. You should eat a variety of fruits and vegetables daily to obtain various vitamins and minerals.

Exchanges/Choices
1/2 Starch
1/2 Fat

Calories 65
  Calories from Fat 20
Total Fat .... 2.5 g
  Saturated Fat .... 0.3 g
  Trans Fat .... 0 g
Cholesterol .... 0 mg
Sodium .... 50 mg
Total Carbohydrate ...... 8 g
  Dietary Fiber .... 3 g
  Sugars .... 3 g
Protein .... 3 g

SAUTÉED ZUCCHINI

Serves 6 • Serving Size: 1/2 cup • Prep Time: 5 minutes

1 Tbsp olive oil

3 medium zucchini, sliced into 1-inch rounds

1 Tbsp lemon juice

1/4 tsp ground black pepper

3 garlic cloves, minced

1. In a medium nonstick skillet, heat olive oil over medium heat. Add zucchini, lemon juice, and pepper; sauté 15 minutes.

2. Add garlic and sauté 30 seconds or until zucchini is tender.

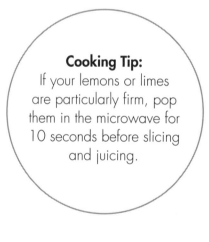

Cooking Tip:
If your lemons or limes are particularly firm, pop them in the microwave for 10 seconds before slicing and juicing.

Exchanges/Choices	
1 Vegetable	
1/2 Fat	

Calories	40
Calories from Fat	20
Total Fat	2.5 g
Saturated Fat	0.3 g
Trans Fat	0 g
Cholesterol	0 mg
Sodium	10 mg
Total Carbohydrate	4 g
Dietary Fiber	1 g
Sugars	2 g
Protein	1 g

SESAME ASPARAGUS

Serves 6 • Serving Size: 1/6th recipe • Prep Time: 5 minutes

Cooking spray
1 1/2 lb fresh asparagus
1 Tbsp olive oil
1/2 tsp garlic powder
1 Tbsp sesame seeds

1. Preheat oven to 450°F. Coat a baking dish with cooking spray.

2. Wash asparagus and cut off ends.

3. Place asparagus in the baking dish, drizzle with olive oil, and sprinkle with garlic powder and sesame seeds.

4. Bake 10–15 minutes.

Cooking Tip:
The ends of the asparagus are usually tough and woody. Be sure to trim them before cooking.

Exchanges/Choices
1 Vegetable
1/2 Fat

Calories 50	
Calories from Fat.....30	
Total Fat ....3.5 g	
Saturated Fat ....0.4 g	
Trans Fat ....0 g	
Cholesterol ....0 mg	
Sodium ....10 mg	
Total Carbohydrate ......4 g	
Dietary Fiber ....1 g	
Sugars ....1 g	
Protein ....2 g	

SPAGHETTI SQUASH WITH PESTO

Serves 11 • Serving Size: 1/2 cup • Prep Time: 15 minutes

1 medium spaghetti squash

Cooking spray

1 cup fresh basil

1 Tbsp pine nuts

2 cloves garlic

1/4 cup light mayonnaise

1 tsp lemon juice

1/4 cup grated Parmesan cheese

Cooking Tip:
This recipe is a quick and lower-fat version of traditional pesto sauce. Pesto sauce has a strong flavor, so a little goes a long way.

1. Preheat oven to 400°F. Cut off the ends of the squash and then cut it in half lengthwise. Scoop out seeds; wash and dry both sides.

2. Coat a large metal or glass baking dish with cooking spray. Place squash halves face down in baking dish and spray the skins lightly with cooking spray.

3. Bake 40–50 minutes. Scoop out squash meat with a spoon and place in a medium bowl. Discard skin.

4. While the squash is baking; place remaining ingredients in a blender or food processor and puree until a paste forms, about 2 minutes.

5. Pour basil mixture over cooked squash and stir to incorporate.

Exchanges/Choices
1 Vegetable
1/2 Fat

Calories	60
Calories from Fat	30
Total Fat	3.5 g
Saturated Fat	0.7 g
Trans Fat	0 g
Cholesterol	5 mg
Sodium	80 mg
Total Carbohydrate	7 g
Dietary Fiber	1 g
Sugars	3 g
Protein	2 g

the healthy carb diabetes cookbook

SPINACH AND ARTICHOKE APPETIZER

Serves 10 • Serving Size: 2 squares • Prep Time: 15 minutes

1 10-oz pkg frozen chopped spinach, thawed and drained

1 14-oz can quartered artichoke hearts, drained

2 Tbsp grated Parmesan cheese

1/2 tsp salt (*optional*)

1/2 tsp ground black pepper

1/2 Tbsp dried basil

1/2 Tbsp dried oregano

2 cloves garlic, minced

1 (12-inch) prepackaged whole-wheat Italian pizza crust

1 Tbsp olive oil

1. Preheat oven to 400°F. In a medium bowl, combine the spinach, artichoke hearts, Parmesan cheese, salt (optional), pepper, basil, oregano, and garlic.

2. Spread the spinach and artichoke mixture evenly over the pizza crust. Pour olive oil evenly on top of spinach and artichokes.

3. Bake for 15–20 minutes.

4. Cut pizza into 20 squares.

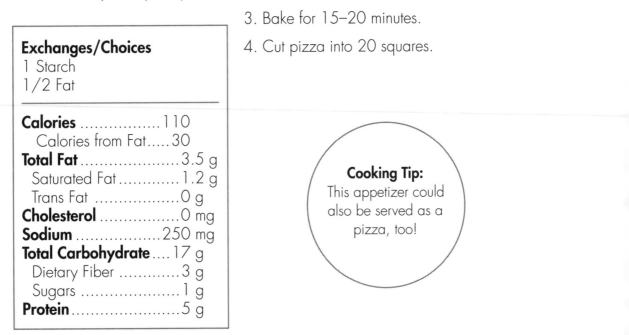

Exchanges/Choices
1 Starch
1/2 Fat

Calories 110
  Calories from Fat.....30
Total Fat ....3.5 g
  Saturated Fat ....1.2 g
  Trans Fat ....0 g
Cholesterol ....0 mg
Sodium ....250 mg
Total Carbohydrate....17 g
  Dietary Fiber ....3 g
  Sugars ....1 g
Protein.....................5 g

Cooking Tip:
This appetizer could also be served as a pizza, too!

SPINACH ARTICHOKE DIP

Serves 10 • Serving Size: 1/10th recipe • Prep Time: 10 minutes

Cooking spray

1 10-oz pkg frozen chopped spinach, thawed and drained

2 13.5-oz cans artichoke hearts, drained and chopped

1 cup nonfat plain yogurt

1/4 cup light cream cheese with chives and onions

1/4 cup light mayonnaise

1/2 tsp salt (*optional*)

1/4 tsp ground black pepper

2 Tbsp grated Parmesan cheese

1. Preheat oven to 375°F. Coat an 8-inch round casserole pan or deep pie pan with cooking spray.

2. In a large bowl, combine all ingredients, except Parmesan cheese, and mix well. Spread mixture evenly in casserole pan. Top with Parmesan cheese.

3. Cover and bake for 30 minutes. Uncover and bake 10 minutes more.

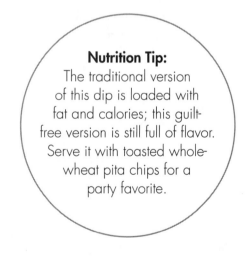

Nutrition Tip:
The traditional version of this dip is loaded with fat and calories; this guilt-free version is still full of flavor. Serve it with toasted whole-wheat pita chips for a party favorite.

Exchanges/Choices
1 Vegetable
1 Fat

Calories	70
Calories from Fat	30
Total Fat	3.5 g
Saturated Fat	1.1 g
Trans Fat	0 g
Cholesterol	5 mg
Sodium	265 mg
Total Carbohydrate	7 g
Dietary Fiber	1 g
Sugars	3 g
Protein	4 g

SPINACH SALAD
WITH STRAWBERRIES

Serves 7 • Serving Size: 1 cup • Prep Time: 10 minutes

Dressing

1 Tbsp + 1 tsp Dijon mustard

1/4 cup + 1 Tbsp balsamic vinegar

1/4 cup rice wine vinegar

2 tsp Splenda

Salad

10-oz bag spinach salad

2 cups strawberries, sliced

1/2 cup slivered almonds, toasted

1. In a small bowl, whisk together dressing ingredients.

2. In a large bowl, add salad ingredients. Pour dressing over salad and toss to coat.

Nutrition Tip:
Not only is this salad a beautiful dish to serve, but it is also full of great nutrition. The spinach is a low-carb source of folic acid, the strawberries provide fiber and vitamin C, and the almonds offer healthy monounsaturated fats.

Exchanges/Choices
1/2 Carbohydrate
1 Fat

Calories 90
  Calories from Fat.....45
Total Fat......................5 g
  Saturated Fat.............0.4 g
  Trans Fat ....0 g
Cholesterol ....0 mg
Sodium ....100 mg
Total Carbohydrate ....10 g
  Dietary Fiber ....3 g
  Sugars ....5 g
Protein.......................4 g

SPRING WALNUT SALAD WITH RASPBERRY VINAIGRETTE

Serves 4 • Serving Size: 1/4th recipe • Prep Time: 10 minutes

1 5-oz bag prepackaged spring lettuce mix

1 gala apple, cored and thinly sliced

1/4 cup reduced-fat goat cheese, crumbled

1/4 cup walnuts, chopped and toasted

1/3 cup light raspberry vinaigrette (bottled)

In a medium salad bowl, toss together salad ingredients. Drizzle dressing over salad and toss gently to coat.

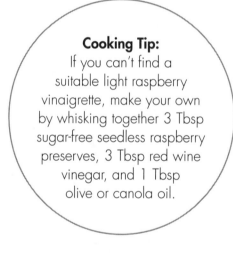

Cooking Tip:
If you can't find a suitable light raspberry vinaigrette, make your own by whisking together 3 Tbsp sugar-free seedless raspberry preserves, 3 Tbsp red wine vinegar, and 1 Tbsp olive or canola oil.

Exchanges/Choices
1/2 Carbohydrate
2 Fat

Calories	130
Calories from Fat	80
Total Fat	9 g
Saturated Fat	1.3 g
Trans Fat	0 g
Cholesterol	5 mg
Sodium	220 mg
Total Carbohydrate	10 g
Dietary Fiber	2 g
Sugars	8 g
Protein	3 g

the healthy carb diabetes cookbook

STUFFED ACORN SQUASH

Serves 8 • Serving Size: 1/4 stuffed squash • Prep Time: 15 minutes

2 large acorn squash (about 2 lb each)

Cooking spray

1/2 green pepper, diced

2 large green onions, sliced

4 precooked turkey breakfast sausage patties, diced

2 slices whole-wheat bread, diced

1/2 cup reduced-sodium, fat-free beef broth

1/2 tsp ground black pepper

1/2 cup sugar-free syrup

Cooking Tip:
If you can't find pre-cooked turkey sausage in your grocery store, buy uncooked turkey sausage and increase the cooking time in step 2 to 7–9 minutes or until sausage is cooked through.

1. Preheat oven to 400°F. Cut off stems on each squash and cut in half lengthwise. Scoop out seeds; rinse and dry each squash half. Spray all sides of the squash halves with cooking spray. Place cut side down in a large baking dish coated with cooking spray. Bake 30 minutes. Remove from oven and set aside.

2. While squash is baking, spray a nonstick skillet with cooking spray. Sauté green pepper, green onions, and sausage patties over medium heat for about 5 minutes. Set aside to cool.

3. In a large bowl, mix together sausage mixture, whole-wheat bread, broth, and pepper. Place a large scoop of sausage mixture into each acorn squash half (divide mixture evenly).

4. Drizzle squash halves with equal amounts of sugar-free syrup. Bake 15 minutes.

Exchanges/Choices
1 1/2 Starch
1 Lean Meat

Calories 145
  Calories from Fat 20
Total Fat .... 2.5 g
  Saturated Fat .... 0.8 g
  Trans Fat .... 0.1 g
Cholesterol .... 20 mg
Sodium .... 240 mg
Total Carbohydrate .... 23 g
  Dietary Fiber .... 6 g
  Sugars .... 7 g
Protein .... 9 g

STUFFED MUSHROOMS

Serves 10 • Serving Size: 1 mushroom • Prep Time: 15 minutes

Cooking spray

2 Tbsp sun-dried tomatoes, minced

1/4 cup wheat germ

3 Tbsp + 1 tsp grated Parmesan cheese

1 garlic clove, minced

2 tsp olive oil, divided

10 medium button mushrooms, stems removed

1. Preheat oven to 400°F. Coat a large baking dish with cooking spray.

2. In a small bowl, combine sun-dried tomatoes, wheat germ, 3 Tbsp Parmesan cheese, garlic, and 1 tsp olive oil. Mix well.

3. Arrange the mushroom caps on the prepared baking dish, cavity side up. Evenly divide the stuffing mixture into mushroom caps. Sprinkle 1 tsp Parmesan cheese evenly over mushrooms. Drizzle 1 tsp olive oil over mushrooms.

4. Bake for 12–15 minutes.

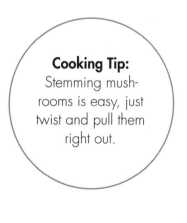

Cooking Tip:
Stemming mushrooms is easy, just twist and pull them right out.

Exchanges/Choices
1 Fat

Calories 50
   Calories from Fat 30
Total Fat .... 3.5 g
   Saturated Fat .... 0.8 g
   Trans Fat .... 0 g
Cholesterol .... 0 mg
Sodium .... 15 mg
Total Carbohydrate ...... 2 g
   Dietary Fiber .... 1 g
   Sugars .... 1 g
Protein .... 2 g

SWEET POTATO AND PARSNIP CAKES

Serves 6 • Serving Size: 2 cakes • Prep Time: 45 minutes

1 1/4 lb sweet potatoes, peeled and cut into 2-inch chunks

1/2 lb parsnips, peeled and cut into 2-inch chunks

1 Tbsp olive oil

1/4 cup wheat germ

2 Tbsp dried chives

1/2 cup nonfat milk

1/2 tsp salt (*optional*)

1/4 tsp ground black pepper

Cooking spray

Cooking Tip:
Roasting the sweet potatoes and parsnips develops the natural sweetness in these root vegetables. Serve them as a side dish right out of the oven.

1. Preheat oven to 375°F.

2. In a large bowl, toss sweet potato and parsnip chunks with olive oil. Spread mixture on a large baking sheet and bake in oven for 40 minutes or until it begins to brown. Remove from oven and transfer roasted sweet potatoes and parsnips to a large bowl.

3. Add remaining ingredients except cooking spray to bowl and mix until thoroughly blended.

4. Coat a large baking sheet with cooking spray. Form mixture into 12 patties and lay evenly on baking sheet. Spray patties with cooking spray.

5. Bake for 40 minutes.

Exchanges/Choices
1 1/2 Starch
1/2 Fat

Calories	125
Calories from Fat	25
Total Fat	3 g
Saturated Fat	0.4 g
Trans Fat	0 g
Cholesterol	0 mg
Sodium	35 mg
Total Carbohydrate	22 g
Dietary Fiber	4 g
Sugars	8 g
Protein	4 g

SWEET POTATOES WITH BROWN SUGAR GLAZE

Serves 9 • Serving Size: 1/2 cup • Prep Time: 60 minutes

Cooking spray

4 large sweet potatoes

1/4 cup nonfat milk

1 Tbsp trans-fat-free margarine

1/4 cup Splenda Brown Sugar Blend

1. Preheat oven to 400°F. Coat a large casserole dish with cooking spray.

2. Wash and dry sweet potatoes and pierce all sides with fork. Place on baking sheet and bake 50–60 minutes, until potatoes are soft.

3. Cut potato in half lengthwise and scoop out meat into a medium mixing bowl. Discard skins. Add nonfat milk and margarine to bowl and whisk until smooth (electric mixer can be used if desired).

4. Preheat oven broiler. Pour potato mixture into the large casserole dish. Spread mixture evenly in dish and top with Splenda Brown Sugar Blend. Broil for 3–5 minutes, until Brown Sugar Blend melts.

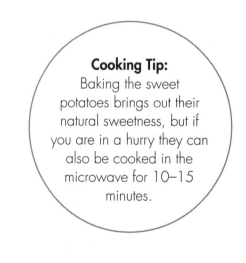

Cooking Tip:
Baking the sweet potatoes brings out their natural sweetness, but if you are in a hurry they can also be cooked in the microwave for 10–15 minutes.

Exchanges/Choices
1 1/2 Starch

Calories 105
  Calories from Fat.....10
Total Fat ....1 g
  Saturated Fat ....0.3 g
  Trans Fat ....0 g
Cholesterol ....0 mg
Sodium ....45 mg
Total Carbohydrate ....22 g
  Dietary Fiber ....3 g
  Sugars ....12 g
Protein ....2 g

VEGETABLE BARLEY BAKE

Serves 8 • Serving Size: 1/8th recipe • Prep Time: 20 minutes

Cooking spray

1 cup quick barley

2 cups reduced-sodium, fat-free chicken broth

1 Tbsp olive oil

2 small zucchini, diced small

1 medium red bell pepper, diced small

1 small onion, diced

1 tsp garlic powder

1 Tbsp fresh basil, chopped

1/2 cup nonfat milk

3 Tbsp grated Parmesan cheese, reserve 1 Tbsp

1/4 tsp salt (*optional*)

1/4 tsp ground black pepper

1. Preheat oven to 375°F. Coat an 8 × 8-inch baking dish with cooking spray.

2. Cook barley according to package directions, using chicken broth instead of water, omitting salt. Set aside.

3. Add olive oil to a large sauté pan over medium-high heat. Add zucchini, bell pepper, and onion; sauté for 5–6 minutes or until onions turn clear.

4. Add cooked barley and sautéed vegetables to a large mixing bowl. Add garlic powder, basil, nonfat milk, 2 Tbsp Parmesan cheese, salt (optional), and ground black pepper. Mix well to incorporate.

5. Pour barley mixture into prepared baking dish. Sprinkle remaining 1 Tbsp of Parmesan cheese evenly over mixture.

6. Bake for 25 minutes.

Exchanges/Choices
1 Starch
1 Vegetable
1/2 Fat

Calories 115
  Calories from Fat 25
Total Fat .... 3 g
  Saturated Fat .... 0.6 g
  Trans Fat .... 0 g
Cholesterol .... 0 mg
Sodium .... 155 mg
Total Carbohydrate .... 19 g
  Dietary Fiber .... 3 g
  Sugars .... 3 g
Protein .... 5 g

Cooking Tip:
Using chicken broth to cook foods like barley and rice gives them a much richer flavor than using plain water.

WHITE BEAN BRUSCHETTA

Serves 10 • Serving Size: 2 pieces • Prep Time: 15 minutes

1 15-oz can cannellini beans, rinsed and drained

1 medium red or orange bell pepper, diced small

1 medium green bell pepper, diced small

1 cup red onion, diced small

1 garlic clove, minced

2 Tbsp olive oil

1/4 cup balsamic vinegar

1/2 tsp crushed red pepper flakes

1 tsp dried oregano

1/2 tsp salt (*optional*)

1/2 tsp ground black pepper

10 slices whole-wheat bread, crusts removed

Cooking spray

1 tsp garlic salt

1. Preheat oven to 375°F.

2. In a large bowl, combine cannellini beans, bell peppers, onion, garlic, olive oil, vinegar, red pepper flakes, oregano, salt (optional), and black pepper. Mix well to incorporate. Cover and marinate in the refrigerator for 20 minutes.

3. Cut bread slices in half. Coat a baking sheet with cooking spray and spread the bread slices evenly on the sheet; do not overlap.

4. Spray the bread slices with cooking spray and sprinkle with garlic salt. Bake for 10–12 minutes or until toasted. Remove from oven and set aside to cool.

5. Divide bean mixture evenly among 20 bread slices and serve on a large platter.

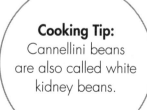

Cooking Tip:
Cannellini beans are also called white kidney beans.

Exchanges/Choices	
1 Starch	
1 Vegetable	
1/2 Fat	

Calories	130
Calories from Fat	30
Total Fat	3.5 g
Saturated Fat	0.6 g
Trans Fat	0 g
Cholesterol	0 mg
Sodium	255 mg
Total Carbohydrate	20 g
Dietary Fiber	4 g
Sugars	4 g
Protein	6 g

desserts

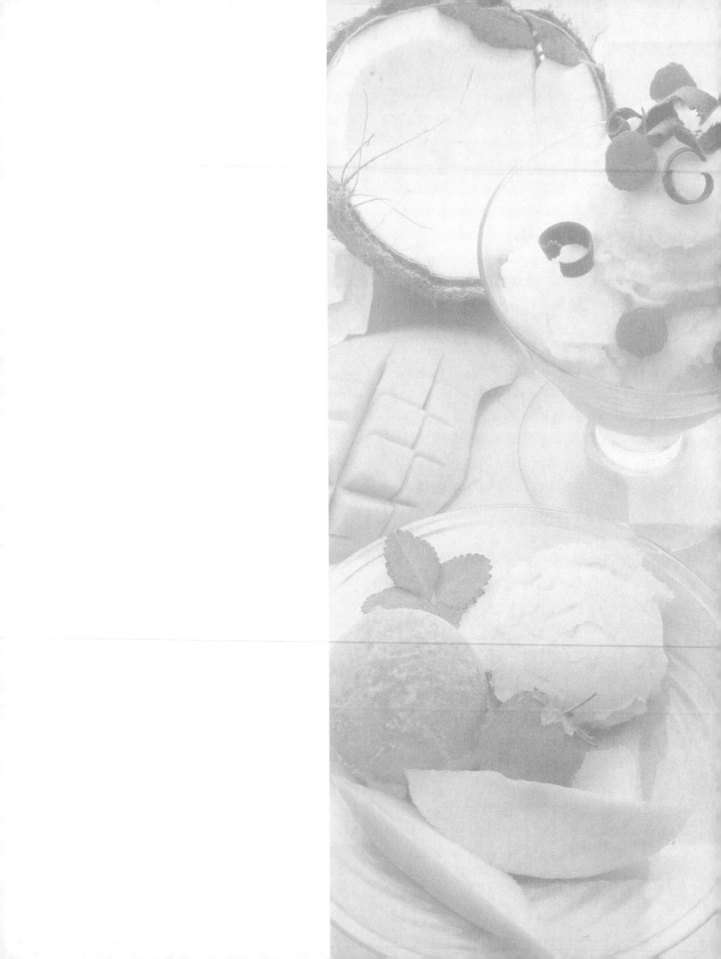

BALSAMIC STRAWBERRIES

Serves 5 • Serving Size: 1/2 cup • Prep Time: 10 minutes

1/3 cup balsamic vinegar

3 Tbsp + 1 tsp Splenda (reserve 1 tsp)

1/2 lemon, juiced

1 cup fat-free whipped topping

1/2 tsp vanilla

16 oz strawberries, hulled and sliced

1. In a small saucepan over medium heat, whisk together vinegar, 1 Tbsp Splenda, and lemon juice. Boil until sauce is reduced and syrup forms, about 3 minutes.

2. Transfer sauce to a cup or bowl and allow to cool completely.

3. In a small bowl, mix together whipped topping, vanilla, and 1 tsp Splenda.

4. In a medium bowl, mix together strawberries and 2 Tbsp Splenda. Drizzle strawberries with balsamic syrup and toss to coat.

5. Divide strawberries into five dessert cups. Top with large dollop of whipped topping.

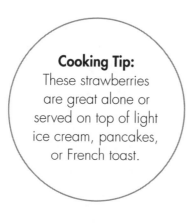

Cooking Tip:
These strawberries are great alone or served on top of light ice cream, pancakes, or French toast.

Exchanges/Choices
1 Carbohydrate

Calories 65
    Calories from Fat.......0
Total Fat ....0 g
    Saturated Fat ....0 g
    Trans Fat ....0 g
Cholesterol ....0 mg
Sodium ....10 mg
Total Carbohydrate ....15 g
    Dietary Fiber ....2 g
    Sugars ....9 g
Protein ....1 g

BANANA BREAD PUDDING

Serves 16 • Serving Size: 1/16th recipe • Prep Time: 20 minutes

Cooking spray
1 pint fat-free half-and-half
2 whole eggs
2 egg whites
1/3 cup fat-free cream cheese
1/2 cup Splenda Brown Sugar Blend
6 cups whole-wheat bread, cubed
1 Tbsp canola oil
3 bananas, peeled and cut into
  chunks
1 Tbsp Splenda
2 tsp vanilla extract
1/4 cup rum (or 1 Tbsp rum extract)
1/4 cup raisins
1/4 cup walnuts, chopped

Sauce
2 Tbsp trans-fat-free margarine
2 Tbsp Splenda Brown Sugar Blend
1/4 cup rum (or 1 Tbsp rum extract)
1/2 cup fat-free half-and-half

1. Preheat oven to 375°F. Coat a 9 x 13-inch baking dish with cooking spray.

2. In a large bowl, whisk together half-and-half, eggs, egg whites, cream cheese, and Splenda Brown Sugar Blend. Add bread and let soak for 10 minutes.

3. In a medium sauté pan, heat oil over medium-high heat. Add bananas and Splenda; sauté for 4–5 minutes. Add vanilla and rum; reduce liquid by half (about 4 minutes). Set aside to cool.

Nutrition Tip:
Trans-fat is found in some margarine products, and it can raise cholesterol levels and increase the risk of heart disease. Read food labels and choose margarines without trans-fat.

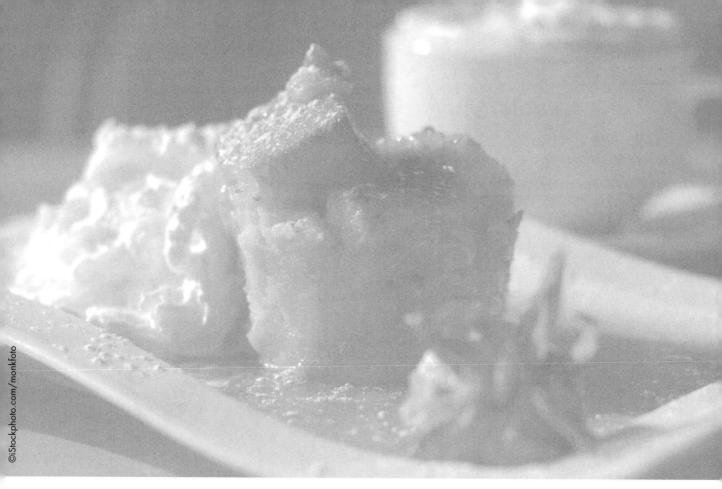

4. Add cooled bananas and raisins to bread mixture, stir gently to incorporate. Pour into prepared baking dish and top with walnuts.

5. Bake for 45 minutes or until slightly firm to the touch in the center.

6. While bread pudding is baking; heat margarine in a small saucepan over medium heat. Cook until it begins to bubble, then whisk in Splenda Brown Sugar Blend over the heat until smooth. Add rum and simmer for 3–4 minutes. Whisk in fat-free half-and-half. Pour sauce over bread pudding after removing it from the oven.

Exchanges/Choices
1 1/2 Carbohydrate
1 Fat

Calories	170
Calories from Fat	45
Total Fat	5 g
Saturated Fat	1.2 g
Trans Fat	0 g
Cholesterol	30 mg
Sodium	165 mg
Total Carbohydrate	24 g
Dietary Fiber	2 g
Sugars	15 g
Protein	5 g

BANANA CROQUETTES

Serves 8 • Serving Size: 1 croquette • Prep Time: 5 minutes

1/4 cup light mayonnaise

1/4 cup plain fat-free yogurt

2 Tbsp Splenda

1/2 tsp apple cider vinegar

2/3 cup peanuts, chopped

4 bananas, cut into halves

1. In a small bowl, mix together mayonnaise, yogurt, Splenda, and vinegar. Place peanuts in a different small bowl.

2. Roll bananas in mayonnaise mixture and then in peanuts. Refrigerate until serving.

Exchanges/Choices
1 Carbohydrate
2 Fat

Calories	155
Calories from Fat	80
Total Fat	9 g
Saturated Fat	1.3 g
Trans Fat	0 g
Cholesterol	5 mg
Sodium	170 mg
Total Carbohydrate	19 g
Dietary Fiber	3 g
Sugars	9 g
Protein	4 g

Cooking Tip:
This is an old Southern favorite that has been made over into a healthy, filling dessert.

BANANA PUDDING

Serves 16 • Serving Size: 1/16th recipe • Prep Time: 10 minutes

2 0.9-oz pkg sugar-free, instant banana-cream pudding mix

3 cups nonfat milk

1 8-oz container fat-free whipped topping, divided

3 small bananas, sliced

1 1/2 Tbsp chopped pecans

1. In a medium bowl, beat pudding mix into nonfat milk with wire whisk for 2 minutes. Let sit for 5 minutes.

2. Fold 4 oz whipped topping into pudding and mix well. Stir in bananas.

3. Pour pudding mixture into a serving bowl. Top with remaining 4 oz whipped topping and sprinkle with chopped pecans.

Nutrition Tip:
Bananas have a higher carbohydrate content than some other fruits. One banana contains 30 grams carbohydrate (2 carb choices), whereas one small apple or peach contains 15 grams carbohydrate (1 carb choice). Only three bananas were used in this recipe to keep the carbohydrate content lower.

Exchanges/Choices
1 Carbohydrate

Calories	75
Calories from Fat	5
Total Fat	0.5 g
Saturated Fat	0.1 g
Trans Fat	0 g
Cholesterol	0 mg
Sodium	185 mg
Total Carbohydrate	15 g
Dietary Fiber	1 g
Sugars	6 g
Protein	2 g

BERRY CHEESECAKE PARFAIT

Serves 4 • Serving Size: 1 parfait • Prep Time: 10 minutes

1-oz pkg sugar-free, fat-free cheesecake pudding mix

2 cups nonfat milk

1 1/2 cups raspberries and blueberries

4 Tbsp fat-free whipped topping

4 Tbsp sliced almonds, toasted

1. In a medium bowl, whisk together pudding mix and milk for 2 minutes.

2. In a parfait dish, layer 1/4 cup pudding and 2 Tbsp berries. Repeat process once more and top with 1 Tbsp whipped topping and 1 Tbsp toasted almonds.

3. Repeat this procedure for remaining three parfaits.

Exchanges/Choices
1/2 Fruit
1/2 Fat-Free Milk
1/2 Carbohydrate
1/2 Fat

Calories 135
 Calories from Fat.....25
Total Fat ....3 g
 Saturated Fat ....0.3 g
 Trans Fat ....0 g
Cholesterol ....0 mg
Sodium ....400 mg
Total Carbohydrate ....22 g
 Dietary Fiber ....3 g
 Sugars ....11 g
Protein.......................6 g

Cooking Tip:
If you can't find sugar-free cheesecake pudding mix, try this recipe with sugar-free vanilla pudding.

BERRY SORBET

Serves 4 • Serving Size: 1/4th recipe • Prep Time: 10 minutes

4 cups frozen mixed berries
2 large oranges, juiced
3 Tbsp sugar-free strawberry preserves
1 cup fresh strawberries, sliced

1. Add frozen berries, orange juice, and strawberry preserves to a blender or food processor. Blend until smooth, scraping sides of blender or food processor often.

2. Scoop out sorbet and serve immediately, garnish with fresh sliced strawberries.

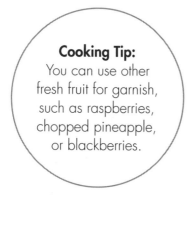

Cooking Tip:
You can use other fresh fruit for garnish, such as raspberries, chopped pineapple, or blackberries.

Exchanges/Choices
2 Fruit

Calories	120
Calories from Fat	10
Total Fat	1 g
Saturated Fat	0 g
Trans Fat	0 g
Cholesterol	0 mg
Sodium	0 mg
Total Carbohydrate	29 g
Dietary Fiber	5 g
Sugars	20 g
Protein	2 g

BUCKWHEAT CREPES WITH BERRY COMPOTE

Serves 15 • Serving Size: 1 crepe + 1 1/2 oz berries • Prep Time: 35 minutes

Berry Compote	Crepes
1 cup blueberries	1 Tbsp canola oil
6 oz raspberries	1 cup buckwheat flour
6 oz blackberries	1 Tbsp whole-wheat flour
1 cup sliced strawberries	1 cup nonfat milk
1/2 cup Splenda	1/2 cup fat-free half-and-half
1/4 cup water	2 whole eggs
	2 egg whites

1. Combine berry compote ingredients in a medium saucepan. Bring to a boil, then reduce to a simmer for 5–7 minutes. Set aside.

2. Whisk together crepe ingredients and let sit for 30 minutes.

3. In a small nonstick sauté pan, pour a small amount of crepe batter in pan, just so it coats the bottom of the pan. Pour off excess. Let cook until edges begin to slightly turn up, about 2 minutes. Flip crepe and finish cooking on other side, about 2–3 minutes.

4. Repeat for remaining crepe batter.

5. Serve warm with berry compote.

Exchanges/Choices
1 Carbohydrate

Calories	80
Calories from Fat	20
Total Fat	2 g
Saturated Fat	0.4 g
Trans Fat	0 g
Cholesterol	30 mg
Sodium	35 mg
Total Carbohydrate	13 g
Dietary Fiber	3 g
Sugars	4 g
Protein	4 g

Cooking Tip:
The first time you flip a crepe is tough, which is why the French say, "The first crepe is for the dog." Try using a spatula to flip up one side and then very carefully pick it up with your fingers and flip it by hand. It takes some practice, but once you get it down, the dog won't get any more crepes!

CHOCOLATE BUTTERSCOTCH TRIFLE

Serves 16 • Serving Size: 1/16th recipe • Prep Time: 15 minutes

1 1.4-oz pkg sugar-free, fat-free chocolate pudding mix
3 1/2 cups nonfat milk, divided
1 1-oz pkg sugar-free, fat-free butterscotch pudding mix
1 8-oz container fat-free whipped topping, divided
8 South Beach Brand whole-grain peanut butter cookies, crushed, divided

1. In a medium bowl, whisk together chocolate pudding mix and 1 3/4 cup milk for 2 minutes. In another medium bowl, whisk together butterscotch pudding mix and 1 3/4 cup milk for 2 minutes.

2. Pour chocolate pudding into bottom of a trifle or medium glass bowl, then top with 4 oz whipped topping and half of crushed cookie mixture. Top with butterscotch pudding, 4 oz whipped topping, and remaining crushed cookies. Refrigerate until serving.

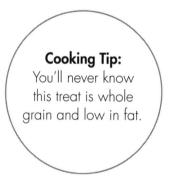

Cooking Tip:
You'll never know this treat is whole grain and low in fat.

Exchanges/Choices
1 Carbohydrate

Calories 85	
Calories from Fat.....15	
Total Fat.................1.5 g	
Saturated Fat............0.2 g	
Trans Fat ....0 g	
Cholesterol ....0 mg	
Sodium ....225 mg	
Total Carbohydrate....15 g	
Dietary Fiber ....1 g	
Sugars ....5 g	
Protein.....................3 g	

CARROT CUPCAKES

Serves 18 • Serving Size: 1 cupcake • Prep Time: 20 minutes

Cooking spray

1/4 cup Splenda Sugar Blend for Baking

1/4 cup Splenda Brown Sugar Blend

1/2 cup unsweetened applesauce

1/4 cup canola oil

4 egg whites

1 tsp vanilla

1 cup whole-wheat flour

1 cup old-fashioned rolled oats

2 tsp baking powder

1 tsp baking soda

1/2 tsp salt

1 tsp ground cinnamon

1/4 tsp ground nutmeg

2 cups carrots, shredded

Cream Cheese Frosting

4 oz reduced-fat cream cheese

1/2 tsp vanilla

2 Tbsp Splenda

1 tsp lemon juice

1. Preheat oven to 350°F. Lightly spray a muffin pan with cooking spray.

2. In a medium bowl, combine Splenda Sugar Blend for Baking, Splenda Brown Sugar Blend, applesauce, oil, egg whites, and vanilla; mix well. Set aside.

3. In a large bowl, combine flour, oats, baking powder, baking soda, salt, cinnamon, and nutmeg.

Nutrition Tip:
These cupcakes are a perfect example of a recipe makeover. Whole-wheat flour and oats are substituted to increase fiber, Splenda and Splenda Brown Sugar Blend are used to decrease carbohydrate content, and applesauce and egg whites are used to decrease fat.

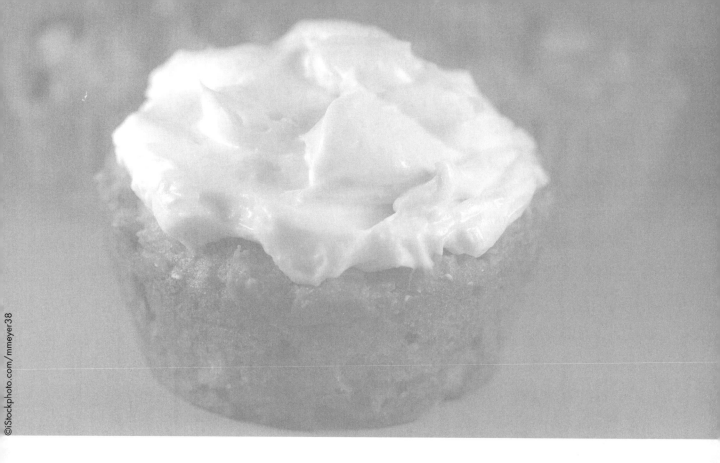

4. Make a well in the center of the dry ingredients. Add sugar (wet) mixture to dry ingredients (all at once) and mix well.

5. Stir in carrots. Fill each muffin tin halfway with batter.

6. Bake until a toothpick inserted in center comes out clean. Let cool.

7. In a small bowl, beat cream cheese frosting ingredients until smooth. Spread a light layer of frosting on each cooled cupcake.

Exchanges/Choices
1 Carbohydrate
1 Fat

Calories 120	
Calories from Fat.....45	
Total Fat ....5 g	
Saturated Fat ....1.2 g	
Trans Fat ....0 g	
Cholesterol ....5 mg	
Sodium ....225 mg	
Total Carbohydrate....16 g	
Dietary Fiber ....2 g	
Sugars ....7 g	
Protein ....3 g	

CHOCOLATE MOUSSE

Serves 4 • Serving Size: 1/2 cup • Prep Time: 5 minutes

1 1.4-oz pkg sugar-free, fat-free instant chocolate pudding mix
1 1/4 cup nonfat milk
4 oz fat-free whipped topping, plus 4 Tbsp
Cocoa powder
4 strawberries, sliced

1. In a medium bowl, stir pudding mix into milk and whisk for 2 minutes.

2. Gently fold in 4 oz whipped topping.

3. Pour 1/2 cup mousse into individual dishes.

4. Top each with 1 Tbsp whipped topping and dust with cocoa powder. Top with sliced strawberry.

Cooking Tip:
Serve this chocolate mousse at your next dinner party—your guests will have no idea that it's lower in fat, sugar, and calories.

Exchanges/Choices
1 1/2 Carbohydrate

Calories 120
Calories from Fat 0
Total Fat .... 0 g
Saturated Fat .... 0 g
Trans Fat .... 0 g
Cholesterol .... 0 mg
Sodium .... 370 mg
Total Carbohydrate .... 24 g
Dietary Fiber .... 1 g
Sugars .... 8 g
Protein .... 4 g

CRUSTLESS CHEESECAKE

Serves 10 • Serving Size: 1 slice • Prep Time: 10 minutes

Cooking spray

1 8-oz pkg fat-free cream cheese, softened

1 cup fat-free ricotta cheese

1 cup fat-free sour cream

2 eggs

1 egg white

1/3 cup Splenda Sugar Blend for Baking

1/2 lemon, juiced

1/2 tsp vanilla

1/4 cup sugar-free raspberry preserves

1 cup raspberries

1. Preheat the oven to 325°F. Coat a 9-inch pie plate with cooking spray.

2. In a large bowl, beat all ingredients (except preserves and berries) with an electric mixer at high speed. Beat until smooth. Pour the mixture into the pie plate.

3. Bake for 45–50 minutes, until golden. Remove from the oven and let cool in the refrigerator.

4. In a small saucepan, melt the raspberry preserves over low heat. Remove from heat and stir in fresh raspberries. Set aside to cool.

5. Remove cake from refrigerator and evenly spread the cooled raspberry mixture over the cake.

6. Refrigerate until ready to serve.

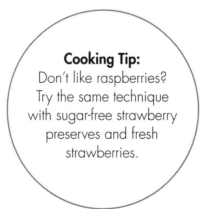

Cooking Tip:
Don't like raspberries? Try the same technique with sugar-free strawberry preserves and fresh strawberries.

Exchanges/Choices
1/2 Fat-Free Milk
1/2 Carbohydrate

Calories	115
Calories from Fat	10
Total Fat	1 g
Saturated Fat	0.3 g
Trans Fat	0 g
Cholesterol	55 mg
Sodium	215 mg
Total Carbohydrate	13 g
Dietary Fiber	1 g
Sugars	10 g
Protein	10 g

GRILLED PEACHES AND ICE CREAM

Serves 6 • Serving Size: 1/2 peach + 1/3 cup ice cream • Prep Time: 10 minutes

1 Tbsp Splenda Brown Sugar Blend

1 tsp ground cinnamon

3 peaches, peeled and halved

Cooking spray

2 cups light vanilla ice cream

1. Prepare an indoor or outdoor grill.

2. In a small bowl, mix together Brown Sugar Blend and cinnamon.

3. Distribute Brown Sugar Blend mixture evenly on the cut side of each peach half.

4. Spray grill rack with cooking spray away from coals or flame. Place peach halves Brown Sugar Blend side down on grill. Grill for 2 minutes on each side.

5. Serve one peach half over 1/3 cup light ice cream.

Exchanges/Choices
1 1/2 Carbohydrate

Calories	105
Calories from Fat	20
Total Fat	2.5 g
Saturated Fat	1.3 g
Trans Fat	0 g
Cholesterol	15 mg
Sodium	30 mg
Total Carbohydrate	19 g
Dietary Fiber	1 g
Sugars	15 g
Protein	3 g

Cooking Tip:
This is a delicious dessert for a hot summer night. You can also grill bananas or strawberries.

ICE CREAM SANDWICHES

Serves 4 • Serving Size: 1 sandwich • Prep Time: 5 minutes

1 cup fat-free vanilla ice cream
8 South Beach Diet whole-grain chocolate chip oatmeal cookies

1. Defrost ice cream in microwave for 5–10 seconds to soften.

2. Scoop 1/4 cup ice cream on bottom side of 1 cookie and top with another cookie. Repeat for remaining three sandwiches.

3. Freeze for a minimum of 2 hours before serving.

Cooking Tip:
Try different flavors of light ice cream for this dessert, like chocolate, mint, or strawberry.

Exchanges/Choices	
2 Carbohydrate	
1/2 Fat	
Calories	145
Calories from Fat	45
Total Fat	5 g
Saturated Fat	1 g
Trans Fat	0 g
Cholesterol	0 mg
Sodium	120 mg
Total Carbohydrate	27 g
Dietary Fiber	5 g
Sugars	10 g
Protein	3 g

KEY LIME TARTLETS

Serves 30 • Serving Size: 1 tartlet • Prep Time: 5 minutes

30 mini-muffin liner papers

Cooking spray

1/4 cup boiling water

1 0.3-oz pkg sugar-free lime gelatin mix

1 cup fat-free sour cream

Juice of 1/2 Key lime

Zest of 1/2 Key lime

1 8-oz container fat-free whipped topping

1. Line mini-muffin pans with liner papers and spray with cooking spray.

2. In a large bowl, stir boiling water into gelatin for 1 minute. Whisk in sour cream, lime juice, and lime zest.

3. Gently fold in whipped topping. Fill each muffin cup about 3/4 full with lime gelatin mixture.

4. Place in freezer for 2 hours. Serve frozen.

Exchanges/Choices
Free Food

Calories 20
  Calories from Fat.......0
Total Fat ....0 g
  Saturated Fat.............0 g
  Trans Fat ....0 g
Cholesterol ....0 mg
Sodium ....15 mg
Total Carbohydrate......3 g
  Dietary Fiber ....0 g
  Sugars ....1 g
Protein......................1 g

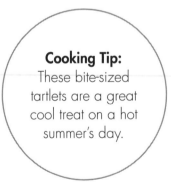

Cooking Tip:
These bite-sized tartlets are a great cool treat on a hot summer's day.

LEMON CURD WITH BERRIES

Serves 4 • Serving Size: 1/4 cup curd + 1/4 cup berries • Prep Time: 5 minutes

1 cup water

2/3 cup Splenda Sugar Blend for Baking

2 1/2 Tbsp cornstarch

2 egg yolks, beaten

1 Tbsp light, trans-fat-free margarine

Juice of 1 lemon

Zest of 1 lemon

1 cup fresh raspberries

Cooking Tip:
You only need a little bit of this rich dessert to feel satisfied.

1. Whisk water, Splenda Sugar Blend for Baking, and cornstarch in a small saucepan. Heat over medium heat, whisking constantly until it thickens.

2. In a small bowl, add egg yolks. Slowly add about 1/4 of the hot Splenda mixture into the yolks; whisking constantly to temper eggs. Pour tempered egg yolks into the pan with the remaining hot mixture over medium heat, whisking constantly.

3. Cook until mixture comes to a boil, continue to whisk constantly. Boil 1 minute while continuing to whisk.

4. Remove from heat and stir in margarine, lemon juice, and lemon zest. Place plastic wrap on surface of curd and refrigerate until cool.

5. Pour 1/4 cup lemon curd into dessert dish and top with 1/4 cup raspberries. Repeat procedure for remaining three dishes.

Exchanges/Choices
2 1/2 Carbohydrate
1/2 Fat

Calories 205
　Calories from Fat.....35
Total Fat ....4 g
　Saturated Fat ....1.4 g
　Trans Fat ....0 g
Cholesterol ....105 mg
Sodium ....30 mg
Total Carbohydrate ....41 g
　Dietary Fiber ....2 g
　Sugars ....34 g
Protein ....2 g

PEACH CRISP

Serves 10 • Serving Size: 1/10th recipe • Prep Time: 10 minutes

Cooking spray

3 Tbsp trans-fat-free margarine

1 Tbsp canola oil

1/4 cup Splenda Brown Sugar Blend

1 1/2 cups old-fashioned rolled oats

2 tsp ground cinnamon

1/2 tsp ground nutmeg

2 15-oz cans peaches in light syrup, drained

1/4 cup Splenda

1. Preheat oven to 350°F. Coat a 9 × 13-inch glass baking dish with cooking spray.

2. In a medium bowl, mix together margarine, oil, Splenda Brown Sugar Blend, oats, cinnamon, and nutmeg.

3. In another medium bowl, mix together peaches and Splenda.

4. Pour peaches into glass baking dish and top with oat mixture. Bake for 30 minutes or until golden brown.

Exchanges/Choices
1 1/2 Carbohydrate
1 Fat

Calories	135
Calories from Fat	45
Total Fat	5 g
Saturated Fat	1.1 g
Trans Fat	0 g
Cholesterol	0 mg
Sodium	30 mg
Total Carbohydrate	20 g
Dietary Fiber	2 g
Sugars	11 g
Protein	2 g

Cooking Tip:
This crisp could also be made with apples or mixed berries, and it would be delightful topped with a small scoop of light ice cream.

PEPPERMINT MOCHA

Serves 4 • Serving Size: 6-oz mocha • Prep Time: 10 minutes

2 cups nonfat milk

4 0.5-oz packets sugar-free hot chocolate mix

1 tsp peppermint extract

1 cup strong brewed coffee

1/2 cup light whipped topping

Cocoa powder, to taste

1. Add milk to a small saucepan over medium heat. Whisk in sugar-free hot chocolate packets and peppermint extract. Let simmer for 2–3 minutes. Do not boil.

2. Add 1/4 cup coffee to a medium coffee mug. Add 1/4 of the hot chocolate mixture, top with 2 Tbsp light whipped topping and a sprinkle of cocoa powder. Repeat for remaining three servings.

Cooking Tip:
Save money by making your own coffee treats instead of going to an expensive specialty coffee shop.

Exchanges/Choices
1/2 Fat-Free Milk
1 Carbohydrate

Calories 120
  Calories from Fat.....15
Total Fat ....1.5 g
  Saturated Fat ....1.2 g
  Trans Fat ....0.1 g
Cholesterol ....5 mg
Sodium ....245 mg
Total Carbohydrate ....20 g
  Dietary Fiber ....1 g
  Sugars ....15 g
Protein ....6 g

PINEAPPLE UPSIDE-DOWN CAKE

Serves 16 • Serving Size: 1 slice • Prep Time: 15 minutes

Cooking spray

1/4 cup + 4 Tbsp Splenda Brown Sugar Blend

9 slices canned pineapple, packed in juice, drained (reserve juice)

1/4 cup + 2 Tbsp Splenda Sugar Blend for Baking

3/4 cup unsweetened applesauce

3/4 cup crushed pineapple

1/2 cup pineapple juice (from can)

1/4 cup canola oil

6 egg whites

1 1/2 tsp vanilla

1 1/4 cup whole-wheat flour

1 1/4 cup oats

2 1/2 tsp baking powder

1 1/4 tsp baking soda

1/2 tsp salt

1. Preheat oven to 350°F. Coat a 9 × 13-inch baking dish with cooking spray. Sprinkle 2 Tbsp Splenda Brown Sugar Blend evenly over pan. Lay pineapple rings in rows of three across over Splenda Brown Sugar Blend.

2. In a medium bowl, combine Splenda Sugar Blend for Baking, the remaining Splenda Brown Sugar Blend, applesauce, crushed pineapple, pineapple juice, oil, egg whites, and vanilla; mix well. Set aside.

Cooking Tip:
Traditional pineapple upside-down cake is made with a lot of butter and sugar in a skillet. This is an easy and higher-fiber version of an old favorite that tastes great.

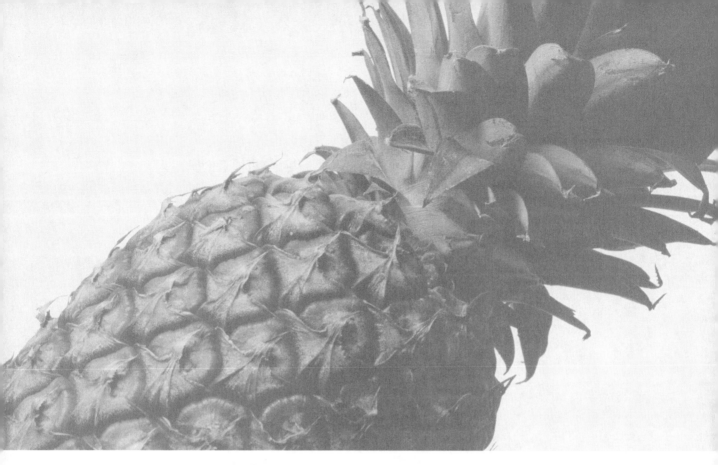

3. In a large bowl, combine flour, oats, baking powder, baking soda, and salt.

4. Make a well in the center of the dry ingredients. Add sugar (wet) mixture to dry ingredients (all at once) and mix until all ingredients are incorporated. Do not overmix the batter.

5. Pour batter over pineapple rings on the baking sheet and spread evenly.

6. Bake 45 minutes or until a toothpick inserted in the center comes out clean.

Exchanges/Choices
2 Carbohydrate
1/2 Fat

Calories	165
Calories from Fat	35
Total Fat	4 g
Saturated Fat	0.3 g
Trans Fat	0 g
Cholesterol	0 mg
Sodium	250 mg
Total Carbohydrate	29 g
Dietary Fiber	2 g
Sugars	17 g
Protein	4 g

POACHED PEARS

Serves 4 • Serving Size: 1 pear • Prep Time: 5 minutes

1 1/2 cups tawny port wine

2 cups water

1/2 cup Splenda

4 Bosc pears, stem on and peeled

1. In a large sauce pot, bring port, water, and Splenda to a boil. Reduce to a low simmer. Add pears and simmer for 1 hour.

2. Remove pears from liquid.

Cooking Tip:
Serve these pears with low-fat vanilla ice cream and a sprig of fresh mint.

Exchanges/Choices
2 Fruit

Calories	130
Calories from Fat	0
Total Fat	0 g
Saturated Fat	0 g
Trans Fat	0 g
Cholesterol	0 mg
Sodium	0 mg
Total Carbohydrate	32 g
Dietary Fiber	5 g
Sugars	23 g
Protein	1 g

PUMPKIN CHOCOLATE CHIP WALNUT BREAD

Serves 16 • Serving Size: 1 slice • Prep Time: 15 minutes

Cooking spray

1/4 cup Splenda Brown Sugar Blend

1 15-oz can pure pumpkin

1/3 cup low-fat buttermilk

1/4 cup canola oil

3 egg whites

1 tsp vanilla

1/4 cup Splenda Sugar Blend for Baking

1 cup whole-wheat flour

1 cup old-fashioned rolled oats

2 tsp baking powder

1 tsp baking soda

1/2 tsp salt

1 1/2 tsp ground cinnamon

1/4 tsp ground nutmeg

1/3 cup + 1 Tbsp chocolate chips (reserve 1 Tbsp)

2 Tbsp chopped walnuts

1. Preheat oven to 350°F. Lightly spray an 8 × 4-inch loaf pan with cooking spray.

2. In a medium bowl, combine Splenda Brown Sugar Blend, pumpkin, buttermilk, oil, egg whites, and vanilla; mix well. Set aside.

3. In a large bowl, combine Splenda Sugar Blend for Baking, flour, oats, baking powder, baking soda, salt, cinnamon, and nutmeg.

4. Make a well in the center of the dry ingredients. Add sugar (wet) ingredients to dry ingredients all at once; mix well. Add 1/3 cup chocolate chips.

5. Pour batter into loaf pan. Top with 1 Tbsp chocolate chips and chopped walnuts.

6. Bake 50–60 minutes or until a toothpick inserted in the center comes out clean.

Nutrition Tip:
Diabetes desserts can still be scrumptious. This bread will be a family favorite.

Exchanges/Choices
1 1/2 Carbohydrate
1 Fat

Calories 145
    Calories from Fat..... 55
Total Fat .... 6 g
    Saturated Fat .... 1.2 g
    Trans Fat .... 0 g
Cholesterol .... 0 mg
Sodium .... 215 mg
Total Carbohydrate .... 21 g
    Dietary Fiber .... 3 g
    Sugars .... 10 g
Protein .... 3 g

PUMPKIN MOUSSE

Serves 12 • Serving Size: 1/12th recipe • Prep Time: 10 minutes

1/2 cup fat-free half-and-half

1 15-oz can pure pumpkin

1/2 cup Splenda Brown Sugar Blend

1/2 tsp salt

1/2 tsp pumpkin pie spice

3 large egg yolks

2 tsp unflavored gelatin

1/4 cup cold water

1 8-oz container fat-free whipped topping

Cooking spray

1. Set a large glass bowl over a pan of simmering water. Add half-and-half, pumpkin, Splenda Brown Sugar Blend, salt, and pumpkin pie spice. Cook until mixture is hot, about 5 minutes.

2. In a small bowl, whisk together egg yolks. Take some of the hot pumpkin mixture and stir into egg yolks to heat them. Once heated, pour the egg yolk-pumpkin mixture back into the glass bowl with hot pumpkin mixture. Heat for additional 5 minutes over simmering water and stir constantly until mixture thickens (make sure to not let the eggs scramble). Remove from heat.

3. In a small bowl, dissolve the gelatin into 1/4 cup cold water. Pour the gelatin into the hot pumpkin mixture and stir well. Set aside to cool.

4. Carefully fold 4 oz whipped topping into cooled pumpkin mixture. Pour pumpkin mixture into a 9- or 10-inch round glass dish (or pie dish). Refrigerate for 2 hours or overnight.

5. Spread remaining 4 oz whipped topping over mousse.

Exchanges/Choices
1 Carbohydrate

Calories	100
Calories from Fat	15
Total Fat	1.5 g
Saturated Fat	0.6 g
Trans Fat	0 g
Cholesterol	55 mg
Sodium	125 mg
Total Carbohydrate	18 g
Dietary Fiber	1 g
Sugars	12 g
Protein	2 g

Cooking Tip:
This mousse could be a great new dessert at Thanksgiving dinner. Your guests will love it!

PUMPKIN SPICE LATTE

Serves 4 • Serving Size: 6-oz latte • Prep Time: 10 minutes

1 1/2 cups nonfat milk

2 Tbsp pumpkin puree

1/2 tsp pumpkin pie spice

1 tsp vanilla extract

3 Tbsp Splenda

1 cup strong brewed coffee

1/2 cup light whipped topping

Ground cinnamon, to taste

1. Add milk to a small saucepan over medium heat. Whisk in pumpkin puree, pumpkin pie spice, vanilla, and Splenda. Let simmer for 2–3 minutes. Do not boil.

2. Add 1/4 cup coffee to a medium coffee mug. Add 1/4 of the milk mixture, then top with 2 Tbsp light whipped topping and a sprinkle of ground cinnamon.

3. Repeat for remaining three servings.

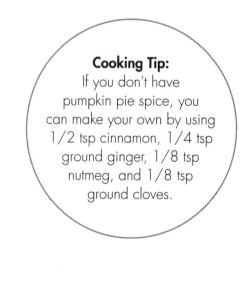

Cooking Tip:
If you don't have pumpkin pie spice, you can make your own by using 1/2 tsp cinnamon, 1/4 tsp ground ginger, 1/8 tsp nutmeg, and 1/8 tsp ground cloves.

Exchanges/Choices
1/2 Fat-Free Milk
1/2 Carbohydrate

Calories	65
Calories from Fat	10
Total Fat	1 g
Saturated Fat	1 g
Trans Fat	0 g
Cholesterol	0 mg
Sodium	50 mg
Total Carbohydrate	10 g
Dietary Fiber	0 g
Sugars	7 g
Protein	4 g

ROASTED PEAR TARTLETS

Serves 12 • Serving Size: 1 tart • Prep Time: 35 minutes

Cooking spray

2 medium pears, peeled, halved, and roasted

4 cups bran flakes, ground in blender

1/4 cup trans-fat-free margarine, melted

1/4 cup Splenda

2 1-oz pkg sugar-free, fat-free instant pudding mix

2 1/2 cups cold nonfat milk

2 Tbsp low-sugar apricot preserves, melted in microwave

1 Tbsp ground cinnamon

Cooking Tip:
To roast pears, preheat oven to 375°F. Coat a large baking sheet with cooking spray; arrange pears across baking sheet and spray with cooking spray. Bake for 25 minutes or until pears begin to brown.

1. Preheat oven to 400°F. Coat a nonstick muffin pan with cooking spray.

2. Slice roasted pears into thin strips.

3. In a small bowl, combine bran flakes, margarine, and Splenda. Press mixture into prepared muffin pan, being sure to go up the sides in an even layer. Bake for 3 minutes. Set aside to cool.

4. In a medium bowl, whisk together pudding and nonfat milk. Divide pudding mixture evenly among cooled muffin cups. Top each with sliced pears.

5. Brush melted apricot preserves gently over pears.

6. Refrigerate, covered, for a minimum of 1 hour or overnight.

7. Lightly sprinkle cinnamon over pears before serving.

Exchanges/Choices
1 1/2 Carbohydrate
1/2 Fat

Calories	140
Calories from Fat	30
Total Fat	3.5 g
Saturated Fat	0.9 g
Trans Fat	0 g
Cholesterol	0 mg
Sodium	405 mg
Total Carbohydrate	25 g
Dietary Fiber	4 g
Sugars	8 g
Protein	4 g

TAFFY APPLE SALAD

Serves 12 • Serving Size: 1/2 cup • Prep Time: 20 minutes

1 1/2 cups nonfat milk

1 1-oz pkg sugar-free, fat-free vanilla pudding mix

1 20-oz can crushed pineapple in juice, drained well

2 cups Granny Smith apples, cored and diced with peel

1/4 cup Spanish peanuts, chopped

1 8-oz container fat-free whipped topping

1. In a medium bowl, whisk together milk and pudding mix for 2 minutes. Add pineapple, apples, and peanuts. Mix well.

2. Fold in whipped topping. Refrigerate for 10 minutes before serving.

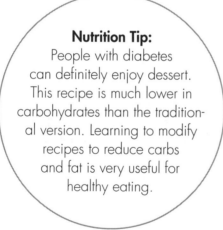

Nutrition Tip:
People with diabetes can definitely enjoy dessert. This recipe is much lower in carbohydrates than the traditional version. Learning to modify recipes to reduce carbs and fat is very useful for healthy eating.

Exchanges/Choices
1 1/2 Carbohydrate

Calories 120
　Calories from Fat 15
Total Fat .... 1.5 g
　Saturated Fat .... 0.3 g
　Trans Fat .... 0 g
Cholesterol .... 0 mg
Sodium .... 150 mg
Total Carbohydrate .... 24 g
　Dietary Fiber .... 1 g
　Sugars .... 16 g
Protein .... 2 g

ZUCCHINI BREAD

Serves 16 • Serving Size: 1 slice • Prep Time: 15 minutes

Cooking spray

1/4 cup Splenda Sugar Blend for Baking

1/4 cup Splenda Brown Sugar Blend

1/2 cup unsweetened applesauce

1/4 cup canola oil

4 egg whites

1 tsp vanilla

1 cup whole-wheat flour

1 cup old-fashioned rolled oats

2 tsp baking powder

1 tsp baking soda

1/2 tsp salt

1 tsp ground cinnamon

1/8 tsp ground nutmeg

2 cups zucchini, shredded

1. Preheat oven to 350°F. Lightly spray an 8 × 4-inch loaf pan with cooking spray.

2. In a medium bowl, combine Splenda Sugar Blend for Baking, Splenda Brown Sugar Blend, applesauce, oil, egg whites, and vanilla; mix well. Set aside.

3. In a large bowl, combine flour, oats, baking powder, baking soda, salt, cinnamon, and nutmeg.

4. Make a well in the center of the dry ingredients. Add sugar (wet) mixture to dry ingredients (all at once) and mix well.

5. Stir in zucchini. Pour batter into loaf pan.

6. Bake 50–60 minutes or until a toothpick inserted in the center comes out clean.

Exchanges/Choices
1 Carbohydrate
1 Fat

Calories	110
Calories from Fat	35
Total Fat	4 g
Saturated Fat	0.3 g
Trans Fat	0 g
Cholesterol	0 mg
Sodium	215 mg
Total Carbohydrate	17 g
Dietary Fiber	2 g
Sugars	7 g
Protein	3 g

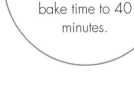

Cooking Tip:
This bread could also be made into muffins, just reduce bake time to 40 minutes.

RECIPES BY ALPHABETICAL ORDER

index

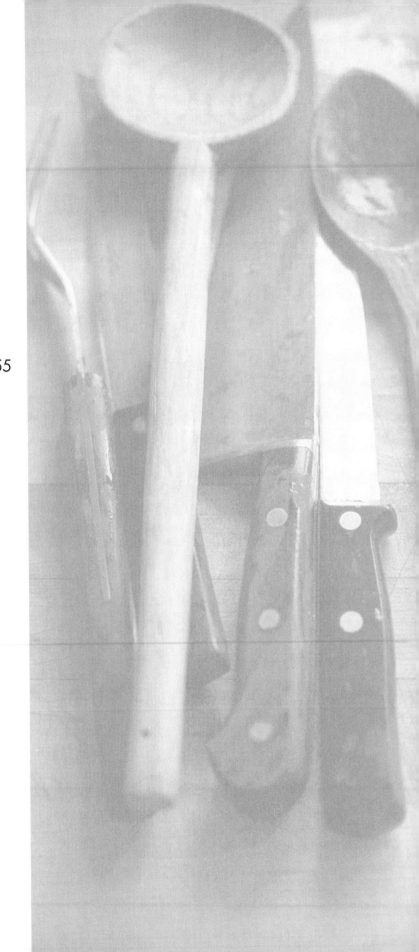

RECIPES BY SUBJECT

Beans

the healthy carb diabetes cookbook

OTHER TITLES AVAILABLE FROM
THE AMERICAN DIABETES ASSOCIATION

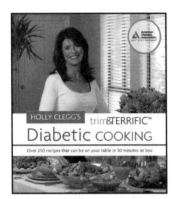

Holly Clegg's Trim & Terrific™ Diabetic Cooking
by Holly Clegg

Cookbook author Holly Clegg has teamed up with the American Diabetes Association to create a Trim & Terrific™ cookbook perfect for people with diabetes. With over 250 recipes, this collection is packed with meals that are quick, easy, and delicious. Forget the hassles of meal planning and rediscover the joys of great food!

Order no. 4883-01; Price $18.95

The All-Natural Diabetes Cookbook: The Whole Food Approach to Great Taste and Healthy Eating

by Jackie Newgent, RD

Instead of relying on artificial sweeteners or not-so-real substitutions to reduce calories, sugar, and fat, *The All-Natural Diabetes Cookbook* takes a different approach, focusing on naturally delicious fresh foods and whole-food ingredients to create fantastic meals that deliver amazing taste and well-rounded nutrition. And absolutely nothing is artificial.

Order no. 4663-01; Price $18.95

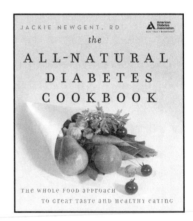

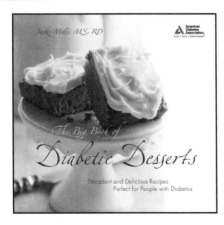

The Big Book of Diabetic Desserts
by Jackie Mills, MS, RD

This first-ever collection of guilty pleasures proves that people with diabetes never have to say no to dessert again. Packed with familiar favorites and some delicious new surprises, *The Big Book of Diabetic Desserts* has more than 150 tantalizing treats that will satisfy any sweet tooth.

Order no. 4664-01; Price $18.95

American Diabetes Association Guide to Insulin & Type 2 Diabetes
by Marie McCarren

Insulin is the most powerful tool available for managing diabetes when pills, exercise, and a careful diet are no longer enough. The *American Diabetes Association Guide to Insulin & Type 2 Diabetes* gives you the complete information on insulin plans you need and gives you advice from the experts: people with diabetes who use insulin.

Order no. 5022-01; Price $12.95

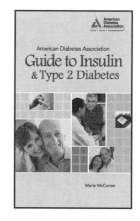

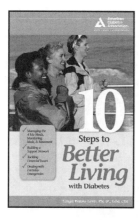

10 Steps to Better Living with Diabetes
by Ginger Kanzer-Lewis, RN, BC, EdM, CDE
Don't let diabetes take control of your life. Instead, take control of your diabetes! Learn the answers to all of your questions about self-care, including the questions you didn't even know to ask. Start living a better life with diabetes—let Ginger Kanzer-Lewis show you how.
Order no. 4882-01; Price $16.95

American Diabetes Association Complete Guide to Diabetes, 4th Edition
by American Diabetes Association
Have all the tips and information on diabetes that you need close at hand. The world's largest collection of diabetes self-care tips, techniques, and tricks for solving diabetes-related problems is back in its fourth edition, and it's bigger and better than ever before.
Order no. 4809-04; New low price $19.95

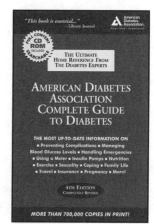

To order these and other great American Diabetes Association titles,
call **1-800-232-6733** *or visit* **http://store.diabetes.org**.
American Diabetes Association titles are also available in bookstores nationwide.